Farewell to Isamu…

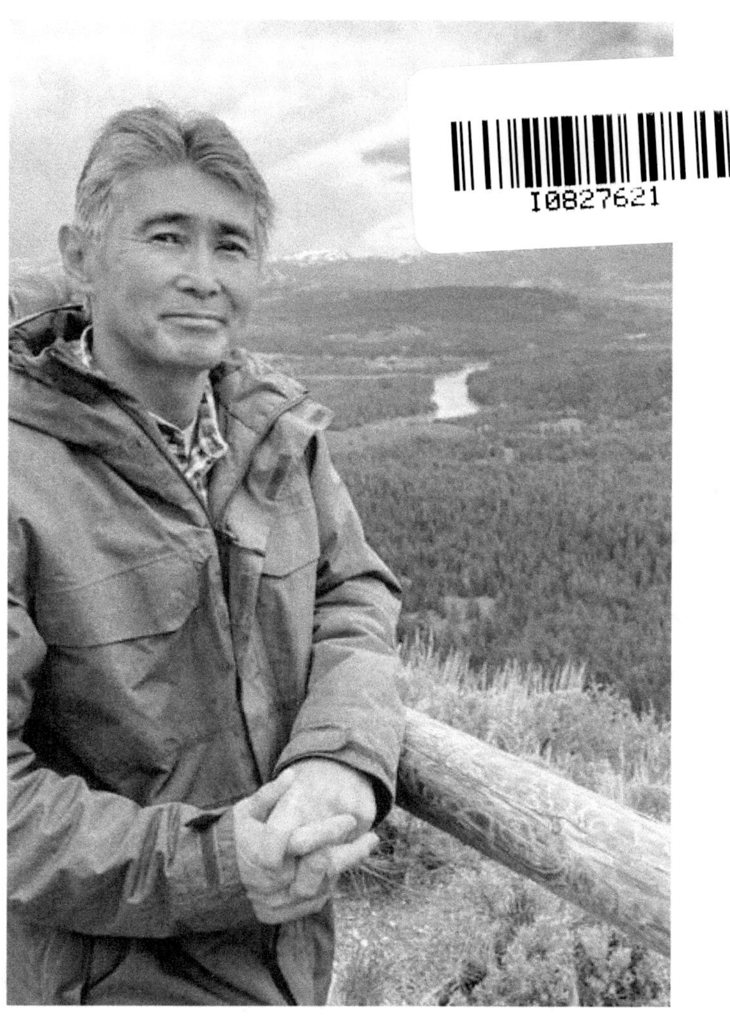

Michael Yanuck MD PhD

ISBN: 978-1-946600-48-6

DEDICATION

In memory of Sam Morishima,
Mentor and friend,
July 13, 1953 – August 14, 2025.

.

"I'm just walking another path in the forest. It's not that bad. It's just another path. So, I would not regret this."
~Sam Morishima.

Dear Reader,

What follows is a written account of my last days with my friend and mentor, Sam, who was the person with whom I made my most significant advances as a Qi Gong practitioner, and who treated me with so much love and support till the very end.

Sam was suffering from a rare and terminal autoimmune condition called Pleuroparenchymal Fibroelastosis (PPFE) that was destroying his lungs. Considering that my prior experiences with Sam had been marked by his medical difficulties pushing me to the limits of my ability in external Qi Gong (and then rising to the challenge!), I was hopeful that this would be the outcome here.

This is the continuation of what actually happened in Sam's final days…

CHAPTER ONE

Tuesday, June 10, 2025

In response to Sam's comments about how his near drowning experience might have thrown off his natural breathing pattern, I said I thought my near drowning experience in the undertow (though not nearly as intense as his) might have left me with similar lingering difficulties: I had this intense fear of not being able to breathe whenever I was in a compromised breathing position, like being in a sauna or sweat lodge; however, I felt that, more than forcing myself to breathe, it would be better to let the feelings come to the surface, then release that retained energy of trauma.

"For me, I practice how to breathe and keep repeating it to properly breathe at my belly and time it," Sam responded.

I'm sure that's helpful, I commented, but if it were possible to release that retained energy of trauma to achieve natural breathing, wouldn't that be more optimal?

"Oh, I would love that," he responded. "But I don't think that's going to happen right now…"

CHAPTER TWO

Post-Study Long COVID-Qi Gong group
Wednesday, June 11, 2025

Sam attended the group virtually; Rosa was the only former participant from the study who was present with me at the medical center. Working with Rosa, I perceived energy at her upper chakras with my hand from about a foot or two away. As I connected with her energetically, I experienced the activation of the crown chakra at the top of my head.

Because of the way that Rosa had positioned herself against a table on her right side, I'd scanned her and then followed the energy with my left hand.

The path of the energy led me some five or six feet away and then interacted energetically with the area around my Dantian.

Next, I felt energy in my right hand, which was heading back to Rosa, and Qi emission occurred around the lateral aspect of her left leg. And since I was positioned with my right leg, standing not far away, my hand wound up moving between our two legs, and I experienced a feeling of cold everywhere along my leg that my hand was moving, so that I could literally track that cool feeling as my hand moved. It was the first time I had really experienced that since Kishore (and then it was a feeling of muscle relaxation, with no hint of coolness).

Rosa commented that she was having a similar feeling of coolness along her leg and other places, which was unusual for her because she usually experiences a feeling of warmth with these sessions.

"Usually I get very hot," she said. "My body temperature increases. I always feel warm in my hands, but today I was feeling cool on my shoulder, and that was unusual and it was kind of emitting out of my body and it was happening more in the right side of my body. and all of a sudden, I started feeling cool along my legs like a popsicle-kind of a cold, and I thought maybe the air conditioning was hitting me and had just turned on and was blowing on me. It was really intense."

"It's hard to interpret what that may mean," Sam commented. "But at least there was a difference. A Delta. And usually that means that a change is occurring. So at least you're experiencing something.

"I think that prepares us for when we're older, and when we have more limitation in our lives," Sam continued. "And so, by preparing us now, those obstacles in the future, which everyone has to face. We'll be able to breeze through it a lot easier than other people, who never had the opportunity to deal with things like that.

"So, in my older age, I think I'd be able to physically and mentally handle it better, and maybe still be able to move about, because I don't have to go through that learning curve - Because I've accomplished that learning curve now; whereas other people have not, and so for them it's going to be a big shock.

"Like when I see young athletes, and they're accomplishing things like I used to do. And I just look at it and I tell them, 'Enjoy it now, because I'm going to tell you, you start up a family, your life changes and you'll find you can't do those things that you're doing now. So, you better enjoy it. And if you're wise, you'll be able to pace yourselves and still train, so that when you do have to change your lifestyle, you're not totally starting from scratch again or with handicaps. You're able to deal with it and figure things out and get back to a decent level that satisfies you in your older age.

"So, I kind of look at this like maybe it's giving me a chance to prepare for my future a little sooner and allows me to breeze through my future a little bit easier and a bit higher in accomplishments while everyone else is struggling. Because it's a big shock when things change in your body."

As for me, even in my college days, I recognized my injuries in childhood made it so that my physical life was limited and had a premonition feeling that I was walking a tight rope, and sooner or later I was going to crash and burn.

It was among the reasons I knew I couldn't carry the weight of a family with responsible I was responsible for. Because something was going to happen to me and I wasn't going to be able to support them. It's among the reasons that I kept myself relatively separate and alone.

Nevertheless, when my leg injury did occur, it was still a shock.

But through it, I found bioenergy and Qi Gong, and they gave me the sense that I could face the future and handle injury and trauma - Because I had this ready approach to deal with trauma...

Next, we performed a Qi Gong self-practice. Afterwards, Sam talked about his experience.

"My hands expanded to the width of my chest and just stayed there," he said.

He compared my experiences over the past week to his, saying, "You described how you felt like your hands were in a tractor beam. That's not my experience. For me, my hands chose to be here. They want to just stay there. Because it's my chest that's injured. So, there's nowhere else that my hands want to be. It's sort of like you have a pet dog, and the pet dog is injured, and there's really nothing that you can do about the injury but try to make the dog comfortable.

"So, you position yourself next to the dog, and you put your hands on its head, and you rub your hands down its head to the neck and the back, and you stroke the dog, trying to make it feel comfortable. And that you're with him. And that you just want to keep petting and petting, hoping that you can make that dog feel better.

"That's why my hands just stay there. They're trying to work with my chest and move with the rhythm of the breathing - With the expanding and contracting of the chest. To try to help make that chest comfortable.

"So, the hands just stay there. They're not locked there. They choose to be there..."

"Because my chest does feel comfortable when I have my hands right here," Sam continued. "And they're kind of moving and pulsating with my breathing and movements of my chest. My hand wants to just stay there. And I feel like I could've helped my hands there for a long, long time. It didn't feel like they were in a tractor beam. It felt like my hands chose to be there. They felt like they were floating there. They weren't trapped. It was instinct. There was no cognition there. They were just there for comfort.

"The energy that moved with the lungs had a soothing effect. Just like when you're trying to give comfort to your pet dog. You hope that it's a healing energy and that every stroke that you're giving to your dog or cat makes a difference."

I recalled sara saying that petting not only increases the dopamine levels in the dog, but also in the person.

I also remembered tom talking about how it was that he felt "petted" when Qi Gong was performed on him.

"I thought the energy was going through my hand to the rest to the arm to the elbow to the shoulder across the chest, and was helping the muscles there," Sam said. "I didn't feel like there was energy there from my palm to my chest, except through the arm and everything else. It was like the contracting of those muscles that was connecting to my chest, to pull those muscles. But it was so subtle, that it felt effortless.

"So, you could say that there's an energy between the hands and chest, but I think that's masked by the muscles contracting all along the muscular system connected between your hands and chest.

"It's like when I hit a ball with a baseball bat: When you do a really perfect swing, it's very effortless. All your muscles are coordinated and just work, so that the end result is a round bat hitting a round ball squarely and propelling that ball out.

"Or someone throwing a football: So that it's not like energy coming out of your palm, shooting that football out. It's the action of your arm.

"With Tai Chi, we labeled that with energy coming out, and maybe there is? I can't say there isn't. But I do feel my whole arm moving, with my pec's being involved in that, and I think that's what massages my chest."

I commented that I thought this was different from my experience with energy: When I follow the energy with my hands, it's not about being connected with the muscular skeletal system; it's about being connected with the energetic circulation.

"Well, the energy travels through your body," Sam countered. "All the Qi Gong I know, there are certain flowing motions that you can feel the energy flowing through your body to through your toes, through your legs, and into the ground - so that you're expelling the bad energy.

"Or feeling the energy coming from the heavens into your head and through your arms and into your body - That's another connection.

"Just the chi running through your body - I think that's all part of it. I think it has to go through the channels of your body. Originally it might come out from somewhere else, just like when you're taking a breath: The lung is one of the few organs that interacts internally and externally - Because it takes in external air and interchanges it into the internal bloodstream - So that there is something of importance coming in from the outside, moving to the inside.

"And it's also taking the CO2 from the inside and expelling it out into the environment. So, you can relate that to bringing in good energy from the outside.

"But the energy here is biological, whereas with the lungs, it's compounds like oxygen and CO2 - That's my feeling."

And listening to Sam, instead of just perceiving energy externally, I was perceiving it internally, feeling it deeper than I ever had before, particularly in the muscles of my forearms.

And it was interesting, because my thumb, index finger and middle finger were actively full of energy, and here I was feeling energy at the origins (i.e., the forearms) associated with the muscles of those fingers?

"One thing that I think is really interesting about Qi Gong is that it goes further than just muscles and nerves," Sam asserted. "I think it goes down to the cellular level. maybe even working with organelles like the mitochondria.

"Maybe it teaches us how to better activate them properly and in sync? Changing metabolisms that occur within these organelles of the cell?

"And this communication might influence the exchange of certain gases? Or the blood to flow better? Who knows? Whatever it does, it's a healthy movement - A healthy reaction - That causes things to be activated appropriately. And maybe turning off other things, so that they would not be so active, like adrenaline and cortisol?"

"Anyways, these are just thoughts," he concluded. "I don't know if they're right, but these are just feelings that I get that this is the purpose or principles or goals of Tai Chi and Qi Gong - That it helps develop that better than any other physical activity. Yoga is good too, but I have a feeling that Qi Gong helps at a deeper level of the body…"

The internal feeling of energy deep in my muscles continued, now in my shoulders.

I told Sam how it was that ruth made the observation that he seems to "activate me."

Sam described the use of fractionated blood for helping diabetics.

"And then you would have your appropriate healing factors that have been fractionated appropriately for healing on day one and day two, and then the person could help heal from a severe wound where

they need some additional help, rather than just the person healed themselves naturally. Like a contractor building a house from the ground up. So, you have these different layers, and the contractor has to coordinate having the materials at the right time.

"So, what I'm trying to say is, Qi Gong might be doing that, too. Trying to activate various components of your body in a timely manner. And therefore, by doing Qi Gong, you may feel differently as compared to whatever other way you undergo healing."

Yes, it was about getting at the innate intelligence of the body to help facilitate healing where there might be problems - To release retained energy of trauma where that energy might be causing problems…

"I want to acknowledge to Sam that I appreciate your metaphors very much," Rosa commented, spiritedly. "I can feel what you're talking about."

"It's really funny," she continued, "because as you were describing how your hands were activated, and you had that ball going up to your chest, I was having the same experience. And I, too, did not want to stop. I just want to keep going.

"And for me, I was talking about how I had that pain in my chest last week… Well, I felt like that ball was drawing me up to my chest, where I started feeling some of the discomfort, and as I was holding that ball, I noticed that my breathing became more profound. And with that systematic breathing going in and out, I felt my chest pain dissipating. So, there might be some correlation between doing that Qi Gong and activating the energy in your body along with the breathing. I think that the two work with one another.

"And one thing that I noticed about you, Sam, is when you first call in, your breathing is a little labored; but when we're talking and you're going through the exercises, you become very calm. So, it sounds like there might be some activation and something going on with your breathing also. And I think the same thing happens with me."

"I think you're very accurate," Sam responded. "The reason why I like Qi Gong is because it does relax me. It puts me in a very nice state. So that I'm able to deal with my limitations of movement and energy a little bit better. It just makes me feel I might be able to get through the little activity that seems so strenuous."

"I think of Qi Gong as subtle healing," he concluded. "So, it's not going to be anything that drastically changes your life, like an antibiotic that's given to someone with an infection and that works

really quickly. Qi Gong I think makes a very subtle difference; but I think it's longer lasting, and it does help…"

Sam left the call to get some rest. Rosa commented that she felt Sam had more energy tonight than other nights.

"He did," she said. "He stayed on for one hour."

Yes, he wasn't fading, I commented. He was not out of breath. He wasn't struggling to breathe. He wasn't coughing.

I commented, though, that it felt like he minimized the potential effect of Qi Gong. In response, part of me was saying, "That's OK. All that matters is that he gets to that lung transplant. As long as that's his goal, then great." But another part of me says, "Well, I wish he had more faith. I mean, it had helped him in the past."

"Yeah," Rosa agreed. "I was going to mention to him about my rash. You remember that Covid rash I had? I got that rash in 2023. So, I had it for at least a year prior to chi gong. And there was nothing that I could put on it to treat it. But after a few Qi Gong sessions here, I just noticed one day that the rash went away. And I didn't do anything different at all. It just went away.

"And I really believe the mindset controls the body. I really believe that with all my heart. So, I try to keep an open mind to healing. I don't want to put any roadblocks or obstacles there. I just want to accept what I can accept.

"I just feel like if you're close minded and think, 'Oh, that's never going to work', then it's never going to work…"

"Do you think he's lost hope?" Sara asked.

At least he has hope in the lung transplant, I responded.

Sara commented that it sounded like the story I'd shared about Wah and Jun-li.

Thirty years ago, Wah Lee was my appointed Qi Gong mentor when I trained under Master Chou.

He'd died some six months before.

The following was a chapter from my first book, Ethel's Story, in which detailed the story of he and Jun-li:

CHAPTER twenty-six
Wah & Jun-li

I had an unused plane ticket and arranged a flight to the east coast. I called my Chi Gong mentor, Wah Lee, and made plans for a visit.

"So, what about this woman you wrote about in your letter?" he asked, upon picking me up at the Rockville Metro after flying in. "Ethel?"

"It's hard to explain, Wah," I said. "It's like all my thoughts of life and the Universe go from an intellectual exercise to something real when I'm with her."

I hesitated.

"There are many times," I continued, "when I'm with Ethel that I'm reminded of you and Jun-li."

"Yes." His voice trailed off. "Did I ever tell you about what happened at Master Chou's temple when Jun-li died?"

"When Jun-li initiated into Chi Gong," he began, "me and the other assistants performed the HoChi Support technique on her. We formed a circle around her, and transferred our energy to her, one-by-one.

"When it was my turn, I feel a real connection with her.

"After the practice, she came up to me and told me that when other people worked on her she didn't feel anything - Like they were just doing it to be helpful, but, really, there wasn't much there.

"But with me, she said she could really feel something.

"The next day I took her to the Great Falls Park near my house. It was so beautiful. We sat on the rocks and looked at the falls.

"She turned to me and said this would probably be the last time she'd ever be there and wouldn't see it again.

"I held her - She cried for a long time. She talked about the things she was going to miss - Her life - Her family - Her children - And just to be that close to another person was very special for me..."

Nearly a year to the day, standing outside the same metro station, Wah pulled up in his car.

"Mike," he said, full of excitement. "Paul introduced me to a cousin who has pancreatic cancer, and I feel a real connection with her."

We sped through Potomac, all the time Wah talking about his experience with Jun-li.

And something about the way he spoke – his hope and optimism – gave me the feeling that he truly could help this woman...

In the darkened gymnasium a frail and emaciated figure sat in the center of the floor.

Several senior members circled around her.

Looking on, I couldn't perceive her breathing...

"We have two new members," Paul Mok announced after the practice. "Brad and Jun-li. They are coming from upstate New York. Jun-li is staying with Joanne and me. Brad has to go back tonight."

Paul turned to Brad.

"Is there anything you'd like to say to the group before you go, Brad?"

Unlike the rest of us who'd been sitting in a circle, Brad was standing to the side.

He wore a sweatshirt that looked a couple of sizes too big for him and hung off his shoulders like a hand-me-down from an older sibling.

"No," he said, in what seemed a deliberately hurtful tone...

Paul called a few days later.

"Jun-li has some questions," he said. "We thought because of your medical background you might be able to answer them..."

On Sunday I went to Paul's home -

Jun-li was sitting on the couch – her tiny frame nearly swallowed by the well-cushioned pillows.

"So," she said in a haughty tone. "You wanted to tell me something?"

In the faint light that filtered through the windows, the woman who sat before me appeared hard and commandeering.

"Sure," I said casually – though, really, I was thinking, "No, I'm here because Paul asked me. I don't want to tell you anything."

There was a certain feeling of entitlement about her that upset me.

"Yes, she's a very driven person," Wah told me later. "She told me so herself. She said she and her husband have worked very hard to get to where they are and like to have things their own way.

"But some people are like that, Mike. I don't hold that against her..."

I talked about my experience – The cancer vaccine and my injury – Experimental protocols and Chi Gong.

"So, what do you think?" she asked, pointedly.

"I think in Wah Lee, you've found the person who could help you most," I responded.

She looked to the side, and for the first time her features softened.

"My husband wants me to come home," she said. "He says he's found a doctor who is willing to treat me."

Then, her features paled, as though a shroud had been pulled over her.

"I don't want to go," she continued. "But he is my husband. He tells me he made sacrifices for me - That I owe him..."

Later in the week Paul called again.

"Jun-li's husband wants to take her back to New York," he said, "and Jun-li is very upset and says she doesn't want to go.

"Brad is a chemist. Perhaps, because you are a researcher, you can talk to him."

I called Brad that evening.

"I believe in all that!" he said. "If I wanted to, I could take her to the best Chi Gong masters in mainland China! But I've been surfing the Web and found a couple of experimental protocols that combine oriental herbal remedies with chemotherapy, and they sound promising!"

He went on for a long time - I listened feeling there was little I could say.

"Do you agree with me?!" he demanded.

I hesitated.

"I agree with everything you've said," I responded. "Still, I can't help but feel that, just by serendipity, in Wah Lee you've found the person who can help your wife most."

"But the experimental protocols!" he pleaded. "They might work, right?!"

"Yeah, sure," I said. "I mean, time will tell."

He gasped and broke off, then sobbed for a long time.

"Okay," he said, his voice was now calm and out of breath. "I'll let her stay another week."

"But after that," he said, resuming his former hurt-filled tone, "I'm coming down to see her, and I don't care what any of you say!..."

"Her husband came and took her away a week later," Wah said. "I could understand his reasons - She didn't have a lot of time left, and he wanted her to spend it with the children.

"Shortly after they started her on chemotherapy, her liver stopped working. I called and called - But each time her husband answered and told me Jun-li couldn't come to the phone - She was too weak.

"I was at Master Chou's house in California when we got the news Jun-li died. Master Chou told us to make a circle and let the thought of Jun-li enter our minds.

"I was doing this, when all of a sudden, this surge of electricity entered my body through my crown chakra.

"I could hear Jun-li's voice inside me – Saying she was alright – And she was happy – And things were okay.

"I burst out sobbing – Tears rolling down my face – I couldn't stop it – I rolled on the floor, back and forth – The others gathered around me. 'What is wrong with Wah?' I heard them saying. 'Why is he crying? He must feel really bad.'

"But I was happy. I was happy that she was okay –That she was fine."

He broke off.

"After that experience I know there is more than this world.

"I am not afraid of death – It is just another part of life. And the things that happen to people are not by accident – There was a reason I should meet Jun-li."

"Still," he concluded, "I do feel lonely, though…"

"The husband put his hopes in something outside of Qi Gong," Sara concluded at the end of the story, "and it didn't end up panning out…"

CHAPTER THREE

Thursday, June 12, 2025
Qi Gong session with Sam.

The energy coming from Sam's upper chakras felt breezy as they ran against my hand. Rather than perceived at the palm, I was feeling it at the lateral side of my hand and it was so different that I really had to trust that it wasn't something like the tingling of one of my own nerves that I was feeling; however, there was the activation of my crown chakra, so I felt I could trust that this was a matter of connecting with the energetic circulation.

Finally, the energy path took me downwards to the ground in a kneeling position, and I stayed this way for a while, until my head felt pulled up, and then the rest of me was made to stand. Energy went out of my hands but remained by crown chakra and then became active at my third eye.

I asked Sam if anything happened for him?

"I felt it in my diaphragm and in my hands," he said. "It was interesting. I was thinking I would feel things in my chest, but I didn't feel anything in my chest.

"But I think it's interesting… I have this headache … Or had… When all of a sudden, I felt this pressure right where I had the headache, which was on the left side by the front temporal area, and it just popped, and all of a sudden, I felt really good. It was like there was a ball of inflammation there that was causing my headache, and then all of a sudden it burst, and all of a sudden my headache went away."

I wondered if it was a muscular release?

"It could have been," Sam responded. "But it felt like it was internal… That it was inside the skull."

"That was good," he declared. "I wasn't expecting that, but it sure is nice to be able to know I could release that headache pressure."

He talked about where he felt the energy in his hands.

"Right there in the metatarsals," he said, indicating that he felt the energy deep. "Not in the phalanges – More in the palms."

He seemed disappointed that he didn't feel the energy in his chest. I asked him to consider that the chi knows what to do and was prioritizing what he needed and was working that way, even if he thought it should attend other needs, like those in his chest. Just like catalyzing that reverse demolition.

I shared my thoughts from yesterday when he made those comments about how the drowning experience might have it affected his breathing, and said that I thought I might be messed up that way, too, from my drowning experience in the undertow, which wasn't near as intense as his, but did leave me somewhat messed up, such that I had this intense fear of not being able to breathe whenever I was in a compromise position, like being in a sauna or sweat lodge, and feeling like, more than forcing myself to breathe, it would be better to get out the route of the illness and release that retained energy of trauma associated with the incident.

"For me, practicing how to breathe and keep repeating it to properly breathe at my belly and time it," he said, fighting through breathing difficulty.

I asked if he imagined it could be possible to let the body lead, so to release the retained energy of trauma, and the body just did it naturally?

"Oh, I would love that," he responded. "But I don't think that's going to happen right now."

Why not? I thought. You didn't think you were gonna have this release in your head, either, to improve your headache.

"What if it could happen?" I asked.

"Yeah, that's true," he responded. "I'm not leaving that out. In fact, I'm waiting for that to happen..."

CHAPTER FOUR

Friday, June 13, 2025
BioEnerQi treatment

Sam lamented about direction of the country.

"So many things are going wrong," he said. "It's layer upon layer upon layer. There was a time that the people in my life were competent. I was always the weak link, whereas all my friends seemed like they were very good at what they were doing. I could always depend on them. And now, it's reversed and it seems like all the people around me are the weak link, so I can't depend on many people.

"It's hard to find very good people who are proud of their profession and their talents. It seems like so many people go for mediocrity and disguise it as competence. People want things from me, but don't want to work for them. They think they should be given it. It used to be that so many people were competent. It made other people more that way. Now, there's so much incompetence that people don't try to be competent. If they do something sort of correct, they're better than most of the other people around them. So, they think they're really, really good."

During the BioEnerQi treatment, I was 6 to 8 inches from Sam's body and it felt like there were these individual energy jets hitting my hand, separated from each other by some 2 inches coming up from him.

My crown chakra was activated.

Sam commented about his sister-in-law's tendency to take the alternative medicine route over conventional practices.

"If there was a choice between standard or something different, the more exotic it is the more attracted she is to it," he said.

I commented that what I did would be considered "exotic."

"I think you're a bit more pragmatic about taking things on that don't have as much foundation to them," he responded. "You see, the thing is, in my opinion, some of these things that are on the fringe work in certain cases, you just have to know when it works and when it doesn't. And people who do the fringe usually give it too much latitude and give it too much credit. And what it causes them to do also just put a blind eye to other more standard methods that may be the better answer. It's like they're looking for a miracle.

"That's very counterproductive thinking. I don't have a problem going to the fringe, but I need to study and understand it to understand how it could help me. I don't have a problem trying things, as long as it doesn't have an obvious adverse effect.

"And then if you see a positive, then you want to keep marching towards that positive. You don't want to run into it. You just need to cautiously take your steps toward it and see how far it can take you?

"It's like when I used to go backpacking up into the mountains and I was hiking in places that no one had ever gone, or very very few. So, there was no distinct trail. So, you follow animal tracks and you pick your path based on where your destination should be.

"But sometimes these paths could go into obstacles, and the best thing to do is to go around the obstacles then to go straight. And you have to figure out which one is the least dangerous path. And you have to be able to say, 'You know, this path is getting worse. I need to pack up and go back', and then take another path…

Being willing to go back and admit defeat and retrace my steps was never something I was good at. Indeed, it was the source of some of my worst traumas.

"A lot of people, they keep going until they fall off a cliff," Sam said. "They're so headstrong.

"So, to me, going down a line of therapy... Well, there are many crossroads and I can go down many pathways. Which one is the best one and which one ends up at a dead-end and which one leads into a swamp and which one leads into a dangerous ledge? When do you back up? When do you change directions? When do you take a side trip? This isn't much different.

"The nice thing is, with medical things, a lot of times you have a guide… Known as a doctor. And you trust your guide, because the guide has been there before, with other patients. So, if they're very

experienced and very competent, they'll be able to take you through the best path. If you can find a guide that is.

"And then if you find that the guide is not that appropriate, you have to make a decision when to change that guide or follow other guides? And this can be very dangerous, because they're supposed to be a lot more knowledgeable than you are.

"That's how I almost fell off a cliff. Because I decided to take a different path from a friend. I decided, 'This looks like a good path. He is moving pretty rapidly. He's older than I am.' I was following him, and he did tell me to follow exactly behind him. But I thought, 'This is just a shortcut. I can catch up with him real quick.'

"And then I ended up on a cliff, and he actually saved my life. Because I was slipping."

I remembered when I nearly fell off a cliff. I did the same thing while trying to follow Deane and christine - They got ahead of me, so I tried to take a shortcut and nearly fell off a cliff.

"It was a good 50, 60-foot drop," Sam continued. "I remember his arm reaching out and pulling him. He was really good."

"Anyway, sometimes you have a guide who sees clearly through certain paths, and other times that guide might not be the best," Sam continued. "In my journey, you don't always walk a path with someone all the way. Sometimes you have to stop and get trained. For example, you're going on a journey, but now you need mountain climbing skills, so what you do, if you take a side path, get some mountain climbing skills, and then go back onto your path. Now, you're able to be more prepared for your journey.

"Or maybe run into an ice cliff, so you have to learn how to climb an ice cliff, using ice pics, and clamps, and all kinds of other stuff. And what you do is, you take a side road, and you get trained on it. Then you get back on your climb.

"Or you have to cross a desert. So, then you have to learn how to survive in a desert environment. So, you go check out someone who knows how to survive in a desert and learn from them and then you go back on your path.

"I see that, like with you, you're getting me through a certain patch that I'm not familiar with. Because you're not going to heal my lungs, but you're going to help me get through a section of my journey.

"But right now it takes up too much energy, as all I can do is hobble along. Everybody has their place in helping me to weather my journey.

"That's why I like these different doctors. The physical therapy helps me. The Qi Gong helps me. The Tai Chi helps me. Even the

roller skating helps me in my efforts to help me correct my body, so that I can move through my journey smoother.

"But I think other people put all their eggs in one basket. And I see that as being very, very foolish. It may work, and I pray that it does for them. But it's like saying - 'Keep on buying lottery tickets', instead of going to work…"

As I continued to work with Sam, there was a lot of energy in my hands and head that seemed to be expelling out to the universe.

"Let me put it this way," he said. "In the past, let's say in China thousands of years ago, there were no lung transplants; but there was tuberculosis, there was consumption, and people had to live with their disease. Some people probably lived a very long life with their disease. And they had to live it in the best way possible. And I believe that the development of Tai Chi and Qi Gong was part of it - Part of that process of improving the quality of how people live back then and help them continue to work and contribute - Or else they would have to die.

"So, if you ask me, I think people use Qi Gong and Tai Chi to be able to continue their usefulness as a living person. And it made them part of the social structure. I think they were limited, but in spite of that, I think they were still functional. It would be interesting if you could go back in time Mike and witness this."

I said I felt I had seen it - with Kino and Madison and Tom. Despite having made no promises, I'd seen them essentially get all the way better with Qi Gong, and, personally, I wasn't closing the door when it came to the possibility of that with him.

"Sure, that would be the cherry on top," Sam responded. "Trust me, I'd rather do this than have my lungs taken out of my chest…"

I felt intense energy at my crown chakra, like it was focused down to a single point at the top of my head, so that I felt tethered to an invisible rope to the sky and the universal Chi above. It was that intense.

And my "talons" – thumb, index finger and middle finger - were activated.

The Qi had directed me into a position where I was kneeling with my head down. Then, it directed me to lift my head, so that I felt in touch with the universal chi, with that focused feeling of energy at the top of my head.

I asked Sam what was going on for him?

"Did you see me shake a bit?" he asked.

I hadn't, as my eyes have been closed from essentially the beginning of the Qi Gong interaction.

"It was like my chest was shaking," he began, "and what I realized is sometimes shaking was releasing things out of my body. They do that in Qi Gong, where you just shake. Stand there and shake your arms, legs, and let your heels rock and things like that - To release tension.

"And athletes do that right before they go and compete. You see them on the sideline. They shake. A lot of people think that they're just loosening up. And I think that part of it is loosening up, but it's also releasing tension.

"And so, in the middle of this, my upper shoulders were shaking, and it was like releasing tension, and maybe the bad energy out of my body.

"It was only for a short while, so that it suddenly stopped. This wasn't the only time. There were a couple of other times when you were doing this that I have that same shaking. But this one was a little bit more significant. It was like it was really doing something, and I felt stronger after that.

"And it was in the chest where I felt stronger, which is where I need it to be. I should have mentioned it when it happened."

Yes, it would have been nice to know what I was doing at that time? If it was during that time when I felt that strong beam of focused energy at my crown chakra right there at a point of my crown chakra?

In any event, I was glad that he had an experience that he thought was particularly significant and helpful.

Nevertheless, it was still my contention that everything we had done before, that was probably just a significant, and that this Qi Gong reached into the innate intelligence with a body and facilitated what he needed most, where he needed it the most, when he needed it the most, at the exact dose required.

Just like what he essentially coined when he described the effect of it as "reverse demolition" facilitates the spark to catalyze the rebuilding of the system, and the self-healing of the system where it most needs it, until it gets to a place like the chest, where he's so happy about it.

So, yesterday when it was interacting with his hands and diaphragm, I think it was probably doing him just as much good.

"Sure, I understand," he responded. "And I think you're right. But today it was in the chest."

As for occurring in the diaphragm and hands yesterday, Sam alluded to the Rolling Stone song, "You Can't Always Get What You Want."

"The one that goes, 'You can't always get what you want, but you get what you need'. 'Sometimes you get what you need'."

I was pulled energetically from a sitting position to a standing position, feeling as though I could have been pulled to the heavens by that tethered cord at my crown chakra.

"Sometimes you just can't explain why," he declared, "but it knows what it's doing."

Yes, it was a complete mystery. Utterly mysterious. It just took me sailing out into uncharted waters. I was a complete explorer. What a joy for someone who loves searching.

"It would be hard to categorize all of these things," he said.

Yes, it would be. And, in general, for me, it was just all about the search and exploration. Just being in a mystery is so much fun. This was where I wanted to be - Having these amazing energy experiences.

"I'd say there are fine ways of experiencing something," he said. "Because when something is infinite in number, is it worth categorizing? How do you limit the infinite?"

Why limit the infinite? I thought to the contrary.

But then again, I knew why: To make it practical. Just like the reason why Western medicine was typically a reductionist practice - so that you can compartmentalize everything and break it down and make it manageable.

"Are people infinite?" Sam continued. "I think when you're talking about physicality, it's not infinite. Human being as physical specimens are quite organized. Very organized, actually. It's very orderly. It's limited. And I think we would wish that we're infinite, but, in reality, when you take a cadaver, it's just an organic body."

I begged to disagree: I thought that each of us was composed of so many unique experiences, so that no two people's experiences were the same, and therefore no two people were the same. And where you can be traumatized in any number of unique ways, and at any number of times and moments, then it does seem to me that you're touching upon the infinite.

But that was OK, because the body knew how to remedy that trauma, and would remedy that trauma, as long as you activated those self-repair mechanisms and gave them a chance to work.

And that was what was Chi Gong was about: To optimize the self-repair of the body, so to restore it to optimal function.

"A lot of people have built philosophies around this," Sam asserted. "'What is a human being? Are we built in the image of God?' And yet, we are so controlled by reptilian functions and nerves.

"And so, venturing off to a more spiritual things… Well, I guess you could say souls have personalities. And what about the soul of a psychotic person? Versus is that of a normal person? The distribution of the kinds of human beings is super wide. And so you could pretty much counteract anything that one says. So, I think it's a fallacy to think that a human being is limitless, and, in reality, probably not. That's why I think we're more finite."

Why God might have created one person to be a saint and another to be a sadist, I had no idea. Yes, my experiences have guided me to an unshakable belief in past lives and that we are spiritual entities experiencing the lessons of the universe on a physical plane. But beyond that, I hadn't a clue.

And as for evolving from reptilian species, these reptilian elements permit us programs that let us reboot, rather than rely on our cortex to get lost reasoning our way out of our traumatic experiences.

"That's a happy place to be, Mike," he responded. "Like you say, we have our experiences. But then, our experiences are finite."

"But I guess there is something that's infinite," he added. "And that's our imagination."

If you ask me, our effect on the universe is infinite and held that the butterfly effect is a no-brainer: You can't go through this life without touching other people, so your effect on this world goes everywhere for all time.

"Yeah, but in that wave of people, energy is also canceling; so that when you have all these butterflies, what you do is, you just have a lot of ripples that ripple into a new norm."

I was happy just being another ripple out there and didn't think I would be canceled out.

"Yeah, but I don't think you have any choice," he declared…

"To enjoy something even simple is infinite in itself," Sam conceded. "Even though it may not be long lasting, it is a joy that could be very intense. But so is sadness - And grief."

Then let's hope we had an ability and opportunity to choose, I responded, and we chose joy over sadness…

"Coming back to an ability to overcome a physical ailment," he said. "Utilizing various methods of medicine and Qi and all kinds of other methodologies, like herbs and combinations of chemicals and

physical movements, and all these things… Well, the body is such that it requires all of these things. It requires nutrients. It requires energy. It requires metabolism. It requires movements. Development. Building up. Chemical compounds within the body. A combination of cells working together. Sensory perception. All these things. It's a very complex form."

What if it weren't as complex as all that? I asked, and if we could get the body back to doing what it was designed to, it could fix itself?

"Oh, yeah, when things are working well, there isn't an issue," he responded. "It's when something breaks down."

So you go to the doctor, and pray he knows what he's doing for you, and made the right diagnosis, and given you the right course of treatment, and this reductionist system of medicine (with its finite way of looking at the body) works out for you, and you don't need to regard the body as possessing an individual physiology with needs beyond that of the general physiology.

As for me, I'm about this energy medicine practice, attending the unique traumas and individual physiology of the body in a way that was guided by that person's innate intelligence; because I think that person's body knows what it needs, and you can get at it via this practice.

"I think you need to keep it simple," Sam affirmed. "The simplest answer is usually the most correct."

"I think you're right, Mike," he added. "I think you're approach is really accurate. If you get bogged down by too many details, I think you missed the picture of what's really needed. I think that's something that you repeated quite often. And it gives you what you need. And you're right: I think everything you've said is very, very correct. I just like to explore the infinite. It's just entertaining for me. And it gives me peace of mind. So, I think it keeps opening doors for me.

"And I think one has to have a reason to live. And the reason for me to live is always that I keep learning something. And it's exciting.

"What I am afraid of is losing the ability to keep grasping things."

Yeah, my father's condition, I thought. At this point, he couldn't hold on to a thought for longer than ten seconds.

"And you know one thing that I feel?" he continued. "It's that learning something and losing that knowledge and gaining it again and losing it, gaining it, repetitively… There's a magic in that, too.

"Because I used to be frustrated. But then, when I learn it again, I'd see something deeper in it - and it's a whole world. I didn't know that this knowledge was connected with this and that, and it starts to

form a fabric of life, rather than the knowledge itself being singular. It's part of the fabric of life."

"So, I'd like to learn something and lose it," Sam declared. "Because when I learn it again, it has a better fit. And being able to grasp and get a deeper understanding of things is very exciting."

At that moment, the energy of the universe was surrounding me and lifting me from the crown chakra, so that experiences like this were about the most exciting things for me, perhaps all I needed.

"That's really good," he said. "That's why you'll be specialized in that area, and I'm specialized in my area."

"And that's the neat thing," he continued, spiritedly "The diversity of people. Because what makes me happy doesn't make other people happy. They have their own happiness. And they need to find that. And I think that just happens without even searching for it. I think people are happy in their own ways is what I'm saying. That's why I think each person is just a part of that fabric of life. One person is no better, no worse than another."

Yes, just another creation of God. Thank God each has their own purpose - So we don't always have to compete with each other and claw away at each other for the same position. Thank God, we were all unique in that fabric. Thank God.

"And what happens when a planet is destroyed? Sucked into the sun, and all the people parish? Will another planet that's inhabited with similar, but not quite the same, receive the same knowledge, and the universe keep on recycling itself?..."

"I haven't had thoughts or a conversation like this in a long time," Sam commented, lightheartedly. "Do you have any pot with you?... That's when it really gets deep."

Sam talked about how he and his buddies would get high on pot and have philosophical discussions about worlds within fingernail clippings?

"High school," he said.

He talked about going to a Led Zeppelin concert at the LA Forum with his high school buddies, in which he served as designated driver, while they got high on LSD.

"Specifically, 'Window Pane' which was LSD crystallized to made to look like a contact lens and applied to the eye," he explained. "You get this tremendous high. My friends were on it in the backseat, and I was driving, because I didn't do things like that. And we got pulled over by a police officer, because a taillight was out or something, and I was giving him my driver's license, and the officer was looking into the car, and my friends were just laughing

and laughing and cracking up. So, the police officer looks at us, and says, 'I'm not going to give you a ticket, but you need to get that fixed. It looks like your friends are having a good time.' This was at the early stages of drugs use, so he just thought my friends were laughing at me getting a ticket. And so, the police officer let us go.

"The concert was canceled because Jimmy Page had hurt his finger, and so we had to ride back up.

"But it was delayed, so our tickets were good. And when we were drove back that second time, it was a phenomenal concert. I'll tell you, there was so much marijuana there, the whole place was full of smoke.

"But that was the most awesome concert, especially when they did Stairway to Heaven. There was a light beam from the ceiling that hit Robert Plant's golden hair, so it was just like really magical."

"So, anyways, those were my friends," he concluded. "We would have all kinds of discussions about life and Pizza. That's how important pizza was as a food choice. I think that's all they ever ordered…"

"Hey, Mike, I appreciate this," he said. "I feel so much better. Please take my words with a grain of salt."

I was about to leave when May invited me for "round two" of dinner, consisting of marionberry pie dessert. She heated my slice and added cheese on top, and Sam had the same...

CHAPTER FIVE

Saturday, June 14, 2025

Before leaving for my father's in Carson City, I stopped at Sam's and performed Qi Gong practice.

This would be the last time I'd see him before that he underwent lung transplant evaluation at Stanford, which was an extensive process to determine not only if he could safely undergo transplantation, but also adhere to strict post-operative care. Hence, it involved not only medical assessments, but psychological ones, as well.

Performing external Qi Gong, the energy from Sam went off my middle finger of my right hand along the lateral aspect and blew my hand upwards until it intersected with the energy coming from my crown chakra, which then felt much stronger.

"It felt good," he commented. "But nothing beyond feeling relaxed yet."

I had plans to meet my nephew when his plane arrived at the Reno airport, so I had to get going, but told Sam I'd miss "camping" with him, like I did the last time he was at Stanford.

"Actually, I'm glad you're not," he said, laughing, "because you've got other things to do. Other places to be. Good books to read. All that kind of stuff. And you gave me literature to read, too. So, I have plenty to do, too..."

CHAPTER SIX

Sam called after meeting with the Transplant team.

"They said I'm going to be deferred," he said. "So, they're taking me off the transplant list. The reason is, my interstitial pulmonary disease, as you know, is a very rare one, and the fibrosis has gone into my chest cavity, so that the lung is adhesing to it. So, for them to perform the transplant and remove my lungs, it's really, really difficult. And would result in lots of bleeding. A tremendous amount of bleeding. So that the risk of survival on the operating table is not good.

"And I could even see that in the eyes of the surgeon who was telling me that. That she did not want to take that risk either.

"But she wants me to complete the testing scheduled for tomorrow. And if it was necessary to do a transplant, they would do it. But then again, they said the cut off was age 73, so, therefore, I have one year, since I'm going to turn 72 next month."

"And so, the chances of getting a lung transplant are slim to none. The only good news is that she said my pulmonary function test is better than it was before, and he said there's some improvements.

"The thing is, the rehab for me is the most important thing, so that it might be able to get me to do a little bit more activity than I currently can do.

"I thought it was important that you knew this, and you're one of the first people I reached out to. I haven't even told my cousin John yet. I will tell him after this. I wanted to let my daughter know first. We just got off the phone.

"Now, I need to find out some really important information, like what is the survival time I have? And what type of quality of life do I

have? And when it's time, how do I go? Do I go slow and painful with slow oxygen deprivation? Do I do it quick and all of a sudden, so I just can't breathe?

"But I don't think they have that information. I don't think they can tell me how much longer? I mean, are we talking months? Or years? I think it all depends on me and how I rehab? if I can stay healthy? I think that's going to be the key thing. Trying to be as healthy as I can. Nutrition, wise and activity wise, and see if I can improve my ability to do things a little bit more. Be able to maintain the basic activities of daily living. Standing in a shower. Moving about the house."

I asked how he was taking it?

"I had this as a backup plan anyway," he responded. "So, it's nothing new. I wasn't surprised. I was hoping that I had better options. I didn't know the extent of how critical or how dangerous the operation was. I thought all the damage was in the lungs, and not the lung cavity.

"But it explains a lot. That's why I've felt like my whole chest strains when I exert myself.

"I was wondering, 'Why is it if it's just my lungs being fibrotic and hardened? Why do I feel this in the cavity of my lungs?' And now I understand why - Because the cavity is attached to the lungs - The fibrosis has extended itself."

"So, now I understand that the pain I feel is because of the scarring. And now that I understand it, I'll try to figure out how to deal with it."

"Anyways, that's the situation, Mike," he concluded. "I tell you, when things are unknown, you don't know what to do. So, you do everything. But now, at least I have a focal point to work on my body, and understand why it hurts, and not be so frightened of it. And maybe I can improve because of that? So, I wanted you to know what I found out today."

I asked if he still wanted to do Qi Gong with me and sara, the way we had planned this Wednesday night?

"I have to do a few other things now, so I better focus on that," he responded. "Because I still need to do a few other things tonight before I go to sleep, and I want to get a good rest tonight."

"But, Mike, I appreciate that," he concluded. "We will do plenty of these things whenever you can do it next. Because this is important to me as well. Even more so now since I can focus on this. And maybe with your knowledge of my situation, we can focus on what we need to work on?..."

Sara had overheard my conversation with Sam.

"It sounds like they feel if they go for the surgery, he'll die," she correctly deduced. "He won't wake up. It sounds like his because his lungs are glued to his chest."

Meanwhile, I was overcome with disgust.

They had the CT, I thought. Why wouldn't the Transplant team have looked at it before bringing Sam all the way back there and putting him through all this? It just spoke of an incompetence that I wouldn't have expected from that institution!

"I hope they're not opening him to stress," sara said. "Talk about 'getting someone's hopes up.' Did they give him any kind of prognosis?"

Sam said he was going to ask about that. I wouldn't be surprised, though, if they didn't just tell him the same thing as those soulless, heartless Pulmonologists.

"Tell him they're just waiting for the next 'step down', huh?" she asked.

Hopefully, they do more than that and tell him about how he's likely to die, which I think will be because of infection.

"Yeah, if he gets Covid, he's probably done," she replied.

If he gets anything, I responded. He has no lung capacity to spare. With that much scarring of his lungs, things get backed up, the bacteria collect, you develop a focus of pneumonia, and that focus grows. He's got no room to compensate. No room for error. No room to breathe. Unless this miraculously gets better, he's just living on borrowed time...

CHAPTER SEVEN

Sam called the next day and told me about the cardiac catheterization.

"It was a long day," he began. "They had some delays, because they had some complications with a patient, so it took a lot longer than expected. I'm feeling a bit dizzy right now, so I'm just going to lie down and rest, but I just wanted to get back to you and let you know that apparently I have a very healthy heart. I wish I could say that about my lungs, but anyways..."

Over dinner, Sara offered her interpretation of Sam's situation.

"If they're telling him, 'You're going to bleed so much that we won't be able to control it', in my mind that translates to he's going to die on the operating table because they can't stop the bleeding," she began. "So, they're saying, 'You have life in you right now. We're going to kill you if we do the lung transplant. If you go under the knife, you're most likely not coming out of it. If you can live with your lungs the way they are, you might as well do that. We can't give you a better outcome. And if you wind up getting worse, maybe we'll do the Hail Mary and fortune will smile on you, and we'll be wrong.'"

"Now, he'll know that he's done everything he could," she concluded. "He's gone to the surgeons, he got the Ooga Booga. Now, he's on the train..."

CHAPTER EIGHT

'Ooga Booga' referred to a comment that my former Qi Gong instructor, Paul Mok, would make at our Qi Gong outreach events thirty years ago.

"A lot of conventional medicine is 'sweet poison,'" Paul would begin. "It makes you feel good, but it plays havoc on the body. It's like the old Ooga Booga joke, which goes like this: Three explorers get caught by a band of aborigines and brought to the tribe's village. There, the explorers are tied up to stakes, and the tribal chief tells them, 'You can choose Ooga Booga or death?' The first explorer says, 'I don't want to die. I'll take Ooga Booga.' So, they take him away and put him through all kinds of terrible tortures until he finally dies. Then, the Chief goes to the second explorer: 'What do you pick? Ooga Booga or death?' He says, 'I don't want to die.' So, they take him away and put him through all these tortures until he dies. Finally, the Chief goes to the last explorer: 'What do you pick? Ooga Booga or death.' The last explorer says, 'I've seen what you did to my two comrades; I think I'll just take death.' The Chief looks at him a little stunned and goes and convenes with the other members of the tribe. Then, the Chief comes back: 'Okay, death it is,' he declares to the last explorer. 'But, first, a little Ooga Booga.'"

Those in attendance laughed, but Paul remained stoic.

"Sometimes, medicine is that way," Paul concluded. "The patient always dies, but the doctor gets to torture him a little first…"

Talking with Sam after he returned from Stanford, at the very least, he seemed exhausted.

"I feel so lethargic," he said. "May drove me home this morning and I took a nap, and I got up, and I felt a little bit better and went over to help John and Stanley, who are still cleaning up the storage unit and dump a bunch of stuff, which was great.

"Letting go of those things has been liberating. They had held me down - Things that I had thought I would need and realize now that I probably won't need them.

"So, it's kind of a relief. Now, I don't have that burden of having to know things and do things. But just taking select a few things that are really more meaningful for the situation that I'm in."

"So, it gives you a focus," he concluded. "And when you have a focus, it's not so burdensome…"

"John brought some peaches for you," he added. "He got it for everybody, but he said, 'Yeah, give some to Dr. Mike.' They are peaches from Fresno, so they're really good.

"Everyone appreciates the stuff you're doing for me and just wanted to show their appreciation.

"Anyway, I have a good heart. They didn't have to put any stents in or anything. No need for stents.

"So, I passed everything, but it doesn't really matter. In fact, I'm debating and wondering if I just should have said, 'Since I'm on the deferred list now, and not on the list for lung transplant surgery, then I shouldn't have to go through the trauma for it.' But I wanted to know about the condition of my heart. So, now I know, and I don't have to worry about my heart.

"I still remember the look on the surgeon's face when she was telling me about my condition. She was very scared about the prospect of surgery. I think she knew that it would be very complicated and even if I got along, my thoracic cavity would be fibrotic.

"Actually, it's kind of a relief. Now I can focus on trying to get myself healthier and try to understand my condition better.

"I did ask the nurse coordinator to try to tell me how long I have and what my progression will be? How long I have to live and all that? She had no answer. I don't think they have much data on it. I guess not everybody is the same, and they don't have somebody like me to compare it with?

"Maybe they'll come up with some kind of medication or treatment that may improve my chances for the future? So, I want to keep that option open? But then again, I only have until I'm 73. That's the cut off for lung transplant."

"Anyway, that's the situation," he concluded. "Right now, my main concern is getting peaches to you before they perish…"

CHAPTER NINE

Last night at the karaoke bar, Sara made a video of my rendering of Barry White's "Can't get enough", and I couldn't resist sharing it with Sam. I told Sam that between singing and dancing, midway through the song I was gasping for breath and didn't know how I was going to continue? Then, midsentence, I thought, "Mike, who do you think you're talking to?" and immediately felt embarrassed.

"I didn't notice that," Sam responded. "I thought you did pretty well... Yeah, you do it very well. And you're really into it. It was really well done. It looks like it was in a pretty cool place to be. Was it in Davis?... You were great. You could see how happy you were."

"I'm so happy that you sent that," he continued. "It kind of cheered me up. I was happy that you were getting some R&R. Because I kind of worry about you, Mike. You kind of stretch yourself pretty thin. I could tell that you were getting rejuvenated. It was like you were a tesla car at a charging station on the fast charge."

I told him, no, and thought it was him that I and everyone else needed to be worried about.

"Actually, I don't want that to happen," he responded. "I just want everybody else to be healthy. Because it's one less thing for me to worry about."

"I think I'll survive, "he added. "I'll survive in a certain way. It's kind of a wonderful challenge for me. Otherwise, this life would be very boring. So, I've just been trying to see what I can do..."

I asked Sam if he wanted to get together, especially as I had plans to fly to Minneapolis for a conference for a few days.

He told me that he was all right, and I should prepare for my trip.

"I'm just trying to gather myself a little bit and organize," he said. "That's what I need to do here for right now. And then I'll see you when you come back, and maybe we'll have some sessions then.

He commented that his dry throat had gotten worse.

"It just seems like nobody understands my condition," he said. "That they can anticipate the things I'm going to go through. Because since these little things that are really difficult. And I think these little things will lead to bigger things."

"But Mike, don't worry," he concluded. "Focus on what you need to do for your trip. I'm sure it will be very fruitful…"

Sam talked about some additional medical testing that had been ordered by his primary care doctor.

"I have to do this and that," he continued. "And I have to fast and some of these fasts are very different. For instance, I can't eat anything for 12 hours prior for one test, and then I can't drink anything for four hours prior for another, and all these things I have to follow so I can just get through to the next thing that I have to do."

That didn't sound very healthy for a patient who could hardly eat? I thought.

"And then people are telling me that I have an appointment for this, and an appointment for that," he continued, "and I'm trying to put those things down, and I'm trying to juggle what I need to do immediately. It's sort of like trying to fight a fire and still planning for long-term reconstruction of the house. And the first thing that you have to do is snuff the fire. But already the people from construction are coming and saying, 'OK, today the folks putting up the walls are coming, and tomorrow the roofers, the next day the window people.' So, I feel like, 'OK, OK, I have to still put out the fire and then get moved in here, so I'm kind of behind and confused, and I'm trying to put things down and grab the paper to put things together.'

"And of course, the coordinator says, 'Here's your visit summary and your appointments for the future', and I go, 'Yeah, but I saw four different people, with four different summaries. Now, I have to put them all together.' And I'm not trying to complain, but this is just the reality, and I have to juggle these things, and that's what I'm doing now. But the demands of the people who are trying to help add a lot more stress sometimes…"

I offered to help with Qi Gong, either face-to-face or virtually.

"Yeah, they seem to both work I think to different degrees," he responded. "But I think with my situation now, I think to myself, 'OK, I have all these different symptoms. How do I focus on Qi

Gong? Or should I not even worry about that and let the Qi Gong focus on me and do what I need?'"

I suggested the latter, with a focus on reversing the scarring.

"Yes, that would be getting right at the source," he acknowledged. "But sometimes you have to trim the leaves before you could see which major branch needs to be cut. And at other times you have to let 'what is' alone and choose the wiser thing to do..."

Sam described regrets about having gone through with the lung transplant testing and evaluations at Stanford.

"That has been going through my mind all this week," he said. "Because I've been asking myself, 'Should I continue on with these tests?' It's like when they told me that the risk was too high for them to do a transplant, I asked myself, 'Well, do I really need to do any more tests?'"

He talked about the problems associated with the cardiac catheterization.

"They told me that the risk of damage was low, but there was damage that was caused by the procedure," he said. "At the time, I decided to go ahead with the procedure for the information that it could offer about my heart. Now, I'm facing the same when it came to the colonoscopy planned for next month. So, I'm asking if it's causing more damage than it's worth? Should I just cancel the colonoscopy, because even if they did find cancer or polyps, that's probably not what's going to kill me. My lungs will kill me first. But then I thought, 'Oh, I should do it. The opportunity is here.' So, I thought, 'I might as well complete it, and just hope that my body is strong enough to recover well and not interfere with a process of trying to become healthier with my situation of the lungs'."

I nodded, just wanting to be a supportive friend.

"That's why it's really important that you let me know your thoughts," he added.

I said I didn't want to push my thoughts on him - He had things that he had to prioritize; but if I could be helpful, I wanted to.

"Oh, yeah, and you have," he said. "You have been and you are."

I confided to Sam that I was concerned that his doctors were just reacting to his illness and not considering the whole picture and how much their tests were taking out of him.

Then, I shared the 'Ooga Booga' joke, then apologized if I'd been insensitive by sharing that story and perhaps it was a mistake?

"It's just that I worry about you, and I don't want you to suffer," I said. "And it's hard for me to not be with you as you navigate the

medical system – because I feel you need an advocate and, as you've experienced, these tests can take a lot out of you."

"But I have very strong opinions," I added, "and this is your life, and I don't want to be a bother or get in the way when it comes to the really difficult decisions you have to make."

"Oh, no, it was no mistake," he declared. "You never made any mistakes."

"No, Mike, you're never a bother," he continued. "And I really enjoyed the video when I saw it this morning. I go, 'This guy has talent.' I went, 'Man, you're a cool doctor.' So, it made me very happy to see you happy.

"So, anyways, don't worry. The point is, you can only do so much. Because you've got your life, and you need to focus on that, and I don't want to feel like I impinged on you.

"You will always be there when I need you, like Qi Gong - You'll provide what I need at the right time.

"So, don't worry about it, you don't have to be with me all the time. You've been with me a lot already and so don't worry. It's like I said, when you start the big juggernaut ball moving, all it takes is a tap to maintain the momentum. It doesn't take much more than that once you got the ball rolling. You did the hard part when you got me moving. Now, all you've gotta do is every once in a while, tap the big ball and keep me moving."

I offered my assistance again when I could be helpful.

"Yeah, we'll talk when you get back. Just do a great job with what you need to do.

"Thanks for your story about Ooga Booga. In the end, it will all be the same.

"Yes, that's what I need to find - What's the best, right path is. It's no different than when I was first born. I'm trying to make the right decisions for my life. This is just another one. I'm still on the mountain, and I'm still climbing up. My options and paths have been limited, and they always are the closer you get to the top. There's always fewer paths that one can take when you get up there. But there are choices, and you need to pick the right one, because the other ones might not get you to the top."

He wished me a good trip.

"I hope that you can find a karaoke bar where you're going," he concluded. "You enjoy..."

CHAPTER TEN

In our weekly "Spirit Buddies" session, I told Steve and sara that I felt Sam had doubts about Qi Gong's ability to help him and wished he would embrace the possibility that it could make a difference to his interstitial lung disease.

"I don't understand that why he doesn't?" Steve said. "Because it has helped him! His experience is that not only did he feel better, But the test showed improvement. The pulmonary test showed improvement. So, that's all the evidence you need. If he's trying to be evidence based, that's all the evidence that he needs.

"Also, the complicating things that he's putting in are not precluded by doing the Qi Gong. He could do those in addition to chi gong. This is really frustrating and must be terribly frustrating for you, because you're offering him health, and he has no reason to reject it - But he is rejecting it. And this has helped already, so it doesn't make sense to me? What do you think is behind this for him? Fear?"

Perhaps at this stage, he feels that what he needs is Western Medicine, because medicines like antibiotics can "cure", whereas it's his feeling that Qi Gong doesn't.

"Too bad," Steve said. "That's really too bad."

And I just had this great sense of cognitive dissonance attached to it, because working with Sam had been the source of my most significant advances as a Qi Gong practitioner. None of my significant successes would have happened had it not been for the work with him. And he was the person who understood my Qi Gong journey more than anyone else. But when it comes to this… Well, he just can't go there.

"I still don't understand," Steve said. "Is he going to some kind

of 'rational' place? Because the evidence says that it helped him. So that's rational. He's just invested in medications or something?

Then, Sara spoke up.

"I understand where Mike's coming from," she said. "But Sam is the one who is dying and he should be given the place and choice to make his own decisions about where he wants to put his energy and what he wants to be working on."

"And as well as being a healer and working with Sam on the Medical Qi Gong, you're also his friend," she added. "You've been his friend for many years. And I hope your desire to give him as much healing as possible with this modality that, at this moment, he seems to not be putting as much emphasis on… Well, I hope that doesn't create a situation where you guys don't spend time as friends. Like I would hate for you to miss out on speaking as friends.

"My experience of being with a loved one who is dying when you can't cure them is that you can walk with them and be there with them throughout the process they're going through. And that's invaluable. That's very meaningful, both for them and also for you when you're left without them. To know that you've walked with them.

"So, I hope that you can balance your desire to try to cure him and alleviate his suffering with your ability as a healer, and not make it so you don't wind up being there for him as a friend…"

I had to get back to my conference; however, as I got off the call, I overheard Steve voice agreement and appreciation for Sara's comments.

"That was very wise," he said, "because Mike obviously wants to do everything that he can, and it's really up to Sam whether he is going to accept what Mike wants to give him or not.

"I also feel that if Mike kind of switches gears and goes, 'OK, I hear you. At the moment, you're focusing on other things aside from Qi Gong and the amazing healing that I can give you. But I am your friend, and let's be friends, and let me track with you as a friend', and maybe that will create spaces in which chi gong can happen, too.

"Whether it does or not is less important than just being there for him. To just stand with him and walk with him through his process and journey.

"I know Mike wants to help as much as he can, but you're absolutely right… The best help that Mike can give Sam is companionship even more than Qi Gong at this point."

"Especially when there's no cure," sara added. "That human connection… That there's somebody there who really cares about

you, and is prioritizing you, and is there for you, and who you can call when you're afraid or when you're in pain… Just somebody who is walking that path with you.

"Because that path of having something incurable and suffering… There is suffering in that path; and having someone who loves you and cares about you and is willing to put their attention on you, I think makes walking that path more meaningful."

"I mean, there's a great amount of medicine in walking that path with someone," she concluded.

"Precisely," Steve affirmed. "And I hope that Mike sees that. He's so focused on what he wants to give Sam, as opposed to just, as you said, 'being there', which is so invaluable..."

CHAPTER ELEVEN

Saturday, June 28, 2025

As I performed Qi Gong with Sam, I described how it was that when I told Jasmine that I was going to Yale, she froze where she stood.

"It was like she was stuck there," I said.

"She was surprised," Sam commented. "She froze. It sounds like she was surprised. It's something that she wasn't expecting from you."

I didn't think I had ever seen that so blatantly in a person, I said.

"So, she was stunned," he responded. "Like all of a sudden, she went from forward to reverse gear. But why do you think she was stunned? Did you think it was because she didn't believe it or think there was a basis for it; and now, you're telling her that you're going to yale regarding your studies, and it gives credence to what you're doing, and she was surprised by that?"

I thought it was because she had feelings for me – and this despite my having given up on pursuing her several years ago.

And I didn't know what to do? Because I was planning to go to yale, and I wasn't staying here anymore. At other times in my life, I'd want to challenge myself and attempt to deal with my feelings when it came to Jasmine and what might be, instead of me just riding out into the sunset and leaving her behind because it wasn't convenient to bring her into a future with me. But now it just no longer wanted to push myself that way - I just didn't want to be vulnerable like that.

"Well, at least there's one thing about you," Sam said. "You're honest, in the sense of your communication. You let everybody know. You're not hiding anything. That's what I noticed compared to other people who hide things and try to manipulate the narrative. You just say, 'Here it is', and let everybody else make their decisions about the situation.

"Other people try to manipulate the narrative to their way of thinking, and don't allow other people all of the information that they need to make a good judgment about the situation. Some people would say you are brutally honest. You're sort of like the person who says, 'I'm going to give you a shot and it's going to hurt - You're going to feel a pinch - You're going to feel a sting - But then, that's it. Versus other people who don't tell you that you're going to hurt, so it has longer-term consequences down the road, because they haven't been honest.

"As long as you keep things honest, and keep letting everybody know where they actually stand with you, I think you'll have less issue of looking over your shoulder.

"You just say, 'This is the situation, and you have a choice'..."

I told Sam that I'd written a letter to Jasmine about this, but wasn't willing to share it.

Sam asked me to consider the possible outcomes.

"I think in your giving her the letter, the best case would be that it would open a door between you two," he said. "The other one would be if she said, 'This guy has it all wrong. He's trying to say that I like him, but I don't have that feeling.'

"If you feel strongly about it, and there's no other consequences for you, then just give it to her. Let her decide. And at least you'll feel you tried."

It challenged so many patterns: In general, when I choose a new path, I would do it alone, without someone I really loved; so, this would represent a change.

"Right," Sam said. "And would this cause more complications? What if she said, 'I'd like to come with you.'"

I wasn't sure. I wasn't sure that I wanted to continue to go into these research projects alone anymore. I did that 40 years ago when I didn't take pebbles with me into my future and, in retrospect, I wonder if that wasn't the wrong thing to do?

"Then you should ask her," Sam asserted. "Give her that letter and see what happens."

"At the very least, you should let her know that you appreciate her kindness, and it felt good every time you got a haircut, and you felt pretty special," he concluded. "I think that's a compliment to her - Make her feel like a person of value..."

As I followed the Qi while performing external Qi Gong with Sam, I was brought to my knees next to him, shoulder to shoulder where he was sitting in the chair, and we were facing in different directions.

And then I felt energy leave my hand, so that I had a feeling of cold and emptiness there, like energy had moved from me to Sam.

For a moment, I was distressed by this. Then, I realized that that was perfectly OK, because the energy would come back to me. That was the pattern. The pattern was that it would just coming back sooner and sooner - Just like it did with Bubble's mother.

Then, I shared with Sam a conversation I'd had with Sara about Bubbles: Sara held that she'd taken the path that Bubbles didn't, by making a life with me when we got reunited.

Sam thought that sara and Bubbles were different, because Bubbles had a child.

I said sara didn't have a child because she made a life with me, instead of going for the other guy, like Bubbles did.

Bubbles could have come back into my life when she had no children, just like sara did. Unlike Sara, she chose not to.

Otherwise, they were pretty similar types - Lovely gentle souls.

And maybe I should honor sara more that she took that road with me that Bubbles didn't?...

Energetically at this point in the session, I had completely recovered the energy loss that I was experiencing in my hand. There was no more feeling of cold and emptiness there. Indeed, there was also an intense feeling of energy at my higher third eye and crown chakra.

"But did you think you ever really lost it?" Sam asked of the energy in my hands. "With a copper wire, you attach your battery to it, there's energy going through the wire. But the wire doesn't change. And yet, through the wire comes power.

"Of course, there was a source at one end, but you could say that the wire was just a conduit. Maybe that's all you are? Maybe the energy comes through the ground or around you, and just like that wire, you didn't change?"

"So, are you the battery or are you the wire?" he asked. "Or are you both?

"They say that chi is like the wind... You can't see wind, but you can see its effect. You see the tree bending over and things blowing, but the wind is invisible.

"But if you are the battery source, then you do get drained. And then, maybe you need a solar panel to recharge yourself? Or some other way to recharge?"

It did feel as though some charge left me, I said.

"Then something had to recharge you," he responded.

Sure, I said. Food. Metabolism. I didn't think it took much to rejuvenate it.

"Open the valve, close the valve," Sam added.

Yes, it was as easy as that.

"You could create it within yourself, this energy," Sam deduced. "Metabolize a meal is to break bonds and transfer that energy."

The point was, there was nothing dangerous or frightening about it.

"Can you be made weak by that?" he asked. "How can one build up that energy, so that you could deliver even more potent energy?"

Who knows? In general, it just seemed that I was getting better at managing chi/energy and related about how it was in medical school, I would become a human torch when frustrated and feel like I'd suddenly "flame on!"

But, in general, that wasn't happening anymore - I think because I'm better at coping with frustration.

"Newton said that energy could not be created or destroyed," Sam said. "It's just transferred. Otherwise, energy is always out there."

The energy of the session was driving my head downward into a prostrate position before my friend, my mentor, my guide.

"Thank you," Sam said. "I feel good. You know, it's funny, I always feel like something has changed when we do this."

I asked him about the possibility of doing this virtually during those times that I had a difficult time getting over to his house?

He indicated that that was fine, especially as he saw me getting busier with my time and needing to be more efficient with it.

"When you make your move, you need to focus on your future, and not my situation," he said. "My situation is kind of set. Yours is fluid still…"

Sam raised the possibility of my staying here.

"Maybe you can establish a clinic in your own home," he said.

Sara had suggested the same, and using one of those office space at Village Homes, where we were currently renting a cottage in Davis.

But I don't want to be a clinician doing Qi Gong. Maybe another time, but not now - Not while I still have the force of will to make more happen, so to advance this practice into the future...

Sam interrupted our conversation to take a call from his mother.

Listening to Sam interact with his mother (Putting her first, and never sharing a word about his difficulties), I thought of the Japanese son from the TV miniseries, Farewell to Manzanar, that my mother held in such regard.

I'd watched the series with my mother in 1976. I could still remember the beginning of the movie when the boats went out, and then came back because war had broke out, and the old Japanese man being questioned by the American officials asking if he could understand the reason why the internment was happening, and the old man responding, "If your mother was fighting with your father, wouldn't you just want them both to stop?"

"Right," Sam said. "That was very profound. So simple, but yet profound. They were just jumping to conclusions that the Japanese people were picking sides."

And then they got to the camps, and the matriarch of the family says to her son, "How are we going to live in this place?" And the son puts his arm around his mother and says, "Mom, we'll find a way. It will be all right." And my mother, who was watching this with me at the time, turns to me and says, "That's how a son is supposed to treat his mother. By being strong and reassuring her."

"Yeah, by offering encouragement," Sam responded.

Yes, and that's what Sam did. Just listening to Sam interact with his mother, I thought, "Sam's the kind of son that my mother would have liked me to have been."

"I'm sure she was very happy with the son she had," he responded.

I wasn't. I read my mother's diary. She would have preferred Sam.

"Sometimes people don't know what they have," Sam responded. "Maybe she didn't realize it, but you were the one who was protecting her at the end there.

"And she might never see all the good things that you did, but you did them anyways. Sometimes the hero never gets the recognition.

Then, he alluded to the movie, "Ford versus Ferrari", and how it was that the driver was gipped out of his Le Mans racing championship.

"He had a clear lead throughout the race," he said. "But the way they measure it. It's not just the person who crosses the finish line 1st, but they add up all the other merits throughout the race.

"When they told him to pull back, the guy said, 'No, this is my chance to prove myself and show the world that I'm the best driver.' But in the end, for the team, he said he would do it. And he backed down and let the other two drivers catch up with him, and they all three finished first. But they gave the win to another driver, because of points.

"And so, he lost the championship, and the title was taken away from him, even though he was the clear winner.

"So, he was very noble to let the other two racers catch up with him, but it sacrificed his win. And he was shocked to find that they didn't give him his trophy.

"What I'm trying to say is, Sometimes noble people, even though they're clearly the winner, doesn't mean that they'll be recognized as the winner.

"So, even though your mother might not have recognized you, you were there; and you did everything that the number one son was supposed to do..."

CHAPTER TWELVE

Monday, June 30, 2025

Sam talked about the nightmares he'd been having during the night.

"It's really telling to me that things are getting hopeless," Sam said. "They're telling me that whatever I do, I'll never get the answer I want, in terms of trying to make myself better.

"It doesn't mean that my dreams are correct; it just means that it's really, really affecting my psyche. I can tell it's eating me away internally."

He described the problems with his throat.

"Last night I tried to drink water to moisten it, but then five minutes later, it would be dry again," he said. "So, I couldn't sleep that night at all. And even when I did, I fall into these nightmares."

"But not to worry, I'm fine now," he insisted. "I'm doing pretty well. Just watching a TV show, and May's been making me some really good food. And having a lot of leftovers. I'm glad we went to the dumpling place yesterday, because that's what I had today.

"That was really good yesterday. I really appreciate your time and effort that you put in. I feel like I'm taking you away from other things, though, that are more important…"

The day before, Sam had shown me a video of Lee Holden performing morning Qi Gong exercises, and now I suggested we do more.

"I would love to do it with you," Sam responded, spiritedly. "The evening one is really good, too. It's totally different from the morning one, which is what I really like. It helps with restfulness and winding down for the day. So, yeah, you let me know when you're in the neighborhood and we'll do it some more."

I asked if it would be OK for me to drive by now?

"Yes, we can do that," he said. "That would be fun…"

Arriving at Sam's, he looked like he was really suffering. He was hunched, his chest caved, coughing.

"How are you doing?" I asked.

"OK," he responded, weakly.

Performing BioEnerQi, the energy took me into a clockwise spin, and I was feeling energy, not only pouring out of my crown chakra (Indeed, it felt like I was perspiring at the top of my head!), but also out of my Dantien; and when I opened my eyes, I was directly facing Sam, positioned on his right side as he sat hunched in the chair.

Earlier, I'd raised the issue of talking with the palliative care folks to give him some ease; now, Sam indicated that he was reticent about reaching out to that service.

"In one moment, I feel like I should be planning for it," he said, "and in another I think, 'Oh, man, I still think I could do something about this. Extend it for a month or a year.'"

"People say you shouldn't give up," he continued, "and I'm still walking. My suffering isn't like someone in deep pain."

It sure sounded like he was suffering to me, I thought, with a shortness of breath and nightmares and difficulties with his throat so that he couldn't sleep.

"All I'm doing is putting a Band-Aid on it," he continued. "But maybe I'll get better?"

He described the nightmares.

"They're really bizarre," he began. "I was driving, and then the next thing I knew, I wasn't driving, and someone was taking me somewhere in a taxi or an Uber; but it was more like a gang that was driving me.

"And then, the next thing I knew, I had passed my destination, so I said, 'OK, just drop me off here, and I'll walk back.' And then they said, 'OK, it's going to cost you so much.' So, I pulled out my wallet, and I had a lot of bills there, and they said it was $18, so I was looking for a $20 bill, and I found a $20 bill, so I pulled it out; but it turned out to be foreign currency!

"So, I go, 'Oh, that's not it.' So, I find another $20 bill, but every time I pull it out, it's a different currency, so that it's Italian or something else.

"And these are gang members, so I'm going, 'If I don't get them the money, they're going to shoot me!'"

"And another time," he continued, "I saw a snake, and I thought it was pretty, so I captured it and took it home. But then, it got away from me, and then it turns into this venomous snake! And I can't find it!

"But then I see it, and I go, 'OK, I need my snake tool (which is a stick with a loop), so that you grab it', but I can't find it. And instead, I find a broomstick. So, I use a broomstick trying to get it. And then I'm chasing it, and I can't find it, and I'm just going, 'Oh, man, my family is going to come home, and I got this poisonous snake, running around the house, and it's hiding all over the place, and there's a million places where you can hide', so that it was a very stressful dream.

"And it tells me that I can't locate the issue in my body, because I keep on getting different issues: My throat, my chest, the problem with walking, and I can't balance very well. I'm losing it. Just like I can't find the snake. And the snake turns from a friendly snake to a deadly snake, and I thought, 'Will this particular illness kill me?'

"And it's just like trying to look for the money. Or trying to get to a certain location: First, I was driving, and then I'm not driving. So, I'm not in control. First, I was in control and able to go to my destination; but even trying to get to my destination was difficult, because I kept getting lost, and all of a sudden, it turns out that it's not me driving, it's someone else; and the person driving is not a friendly person - It's a very deadly person.

"And the thing is, they really don't get me to the place I want to go. But I have to make it work to get back; and then I have to pay them; and I can't pay them.

"And it seems like I have a wallet, and I have a bunch of bills in there; but none of the bills is the right bill. They're totally useless bills. Because the currency is totally off.

"So, in my mind, it's telling me that whatever I do, it's pretty hopeless. I'm not getting the results I want. Not from the exercises. Not from the medicines. Nothing's working. I keep slipping.

"And you're asking me, 'Maybe you need palliative care?' And maybe that's what my dreams are telling me.

"But then, again, the dreams aren't saying I'm dying; It just says I'm having a difficult time finding the right solutions. So, I keep thinking, 'Maybe there is a solution out there still?'

"In one sense, though, I'm just saying, 'I'm getting tired. I can't find an answer. And maybe there isn't an answer'..."

I suggested potentially assuming that perhaps this was all related to one process? Like perhaps this was all related to an autoimmune process? Such that the underlying cause was an immune condition that had gone haywire.

"The worst place that it's going haywire is in your lungs," I contended, "so to produce all the scarring there. But maybe the immune system is going haywire everywhere? This way we could bring it all down to one cause. It was the immune system and an auto-immune process. And this way, perhaps we could do less scrambling and be less concerned about the possibility that there's a different process here and another process there, and could just focus on the one process?"

Sam indicated agreement, saying he had gone to an allergist who had found that he was allergic to multiple antigens.

"Pollen and all this," he said. "Bushes and trees."

He described how all the outpatient appointments had set him back.

"Before that, I could do the Qi Gong," he complained. "Now, I can hardly do it..."

CHAPTER THIRTEEN

Tuesday, July 2, 2025

Sam wondered that, where both Qi Gong and acupuncture were traditional Chinese medicine approaches, if that entitled me to be monetarily reimbursed for my efforts?

I suppose, I responded. As for me, I wasn't looking to be paid for Qi Gong by patients or establishing a Qi Gong practice, I was looking to understand the energetic circulation - The Chi. What is behind all of traditional Chinese medicine. What might be behind all of religion. What might be behind spirituality. What might be behind a connection with the "sacred presence."

Because when it comes to all of these different practices within traditional Chinese medicine, whether they include acupuncture or Qi Gong or Tai Chi or herbs, the basis is always the same - The chi. And yet, we had no way of measuring this. No way of understanding the underlying physiology. Instead, it's relegated to having "no basis in physical reality." That means all of these practices, to date, have no basis in physical reality.

That's my source of difficulty with all this. That's where I get hung up. That's where I asked the question, What is the point of learning all of these acupuncture points if we don't know how they work? To me, it's like designing and putting together an experiment without knowing what the ingredients are.

When it comes to medications, we understand what they're doing at the molecular level. And I want that for traditional Chinese medicine, too - Including and especially Qi Gong.

Sam argued that there were meridians and acupuncture points and a system they follow.

But is that physiology? I asked.

"No, but apparently people have accepted it," he said.

Yes, it was accepted based on the randomized clinical trials that it had been beneficial for a vast number of conditions. But I want to understand it at a physiologic level.

Sam suggested I study acupuncture.

"Maybe it would help," he said.

But it just seemed to me that acupuncture was just another approach that involved blind faith in something that had "no physical basis in reality" as of yet. And I wanted to understand and search for that physical basis. That's my goal.

"But don't you think that it might be a door?" he asked. "And if you opened that door by understanding this a little bit better and understanding the correlation, it could help you in your search for chi?

He asked if my other masters practice acupuncture?

Yes, I responded. Indeed, Master Chou was a licensed acupuncturist.

"You see, he knows both," Sam said. "What does he feel? what a student studying acupuncture be an appropriate person for you to teach she gone? Or are they too biased and want to lay a needle onto the point, rather than do it externally the way you do it?

"Look how biased I was, coming from my bioenergy background," I said. "I think it's OK when it came to people coming from various backgrounds. Hopefully we're all just like blind men feeling at the elephant and trying to put it all together. And hopefully we're all just different specialist trying to understand our peace in this puzzle. And one day we'll put this whole puzzle together.

"I just think it would be nice if you had a way of generating money for your own practice," he said...

On the subject of acquiring money, I shared that Sara's sister was trying to help me acquire funds from a very wealth donor to the sister's research who had recently become extremely interested in Qi Gong, however, the donor was also against vaccines.

Sam didn't think it would work.

"You're very strong with your beliefs," he said. "Really, it's not just about beliefs - You're very strong about the truth. You don't have an ideology. You just have facts. And you go with the facts. And that's not an ideology."

"Whereas with ideology," he continued, "you can't argue against an ideology. It's like the old saying: 'You can't argue against stupid.'

"So, I would say, 'Fat chance.' You could probably fool her for a while, but it would slip - And you know what happens when things slip."

Yes, I said. I hadn't pursued it in the first place because I was concerned I would sink her sister.

"Right," he affirmed...

May invited me to join them for dinner, and Sam, May and I sat in the kitchen and had a nice spaghetti meal.

At the end of dinner, Sam chided that actually I came for May's cooking, rather than perform any Qi Gong with him, and given how often I'd repeatedly said, "Yum," through the meal (which reminded me of the night that I was eating my mother's spaghetti and meatball sauce, and couldn't stop saying, "Yum", so that my mom sent me away from the table), I had to agree...

CHAPTER FOURTEEN

Wednesday, July 2, 2025

I performed Qi Gong with Sam, and it struck me that whereas before I would be imbued with a feeling of awe and reverence, it was more focused, so that I had this intense feeling at my crown chakra? Like the awe and reverence had moved to the crown chakra point as my connection with the divine.

Scanning Sam with my right hand, I had that feeling of being "plugged in", so that just felt like 1000 cables were being shot into my hand like a lot of focused beams or chords of light coming from his chest.

I was standing in front of Sam, although with my body sideways, with my right shoulder, closest to him as he sat.

And I was feeling energy all over me, especially in my shoulders, in a kind of internal way, which was different than the way I usually experience energy.

Then, it felt like I was being moved away from Sam, as though I'd been encased in some energy bubble and slid away from Sam.

This was another new and unique experience. It wasn't like I was following the energy as it was leading me away from Sam - like the energy came and moved me en masse. As though I'd been placed in some kind of tractor beam and then move to the side.

Not long after, the energy left my hand, but there was still energy at the top of my head, and also a feeling of energy at my chest - so that my chest was all full and opened up, which was not my usual state.

There was a feeling of energy between my chest and my right hand…

Qi Gong self-practice virtually with the group from Sam's house followed. My brother had called in to join the virtual session, and we were waiting for the others.

I asked Sam if he was perceiving anything? He indicated that he was not.

This concern me, because it wasn't like Sam to indicate that he had not experienced anything with the external Qi Gong, so I wondered if this venue was just not going to work for him?

I opened the line so that Whitney and ruth could join us virtually over the teams call, then began leading the Qi Gong self-practice.

After about ten minutes, I announced that the energy had left my hands but told the others not to stop if they were still having an energy experience, and, in the meantime, I would tell them about my energy experience.

In my case, at some point, the energy took my hands together to hold that ball of energy and then directed towards my face, so that I could feel the energy from my hands against my face and the cool tingling that it produced, and then it directed my hands down my body, so that I continue to feel the healing energy from my hands everywhere that they came near, especially above my ankles, where I sat cross legged on Sam's couch.

Ruth shared her experience, which she described as different from others.

"I really felt like I had a tornado coming down from the sky onto my heart," she began. "When I first started, I felt that coolness of the energy between my hands, and wherever I move my hands, I feel that coolness on my body."

This was not unlike my experience.

"And then after that tornado came in, I felt like everything changed to hot, and my body was real sensitive to touch, so that when I laid a hand on my arm, it just felt hot. And I tried the other one, and it felt hot, too.

"And my arms were doing a lot of movement. Just both of them really moving around.

"And I was actually standing, which was a different experience, because I've always been seated, but I heard Sam saying that he did it standing, so I decided to try it. And I even felt like I needed to spin for a little bit. So, there was just a lot of body activity with my experience tonight."

It really sounded like ruth had taken a quantum leap in her ability with Qi Gong.

"And it was fun," she added. "I did feel really energized while doing that."

I asked if the feeling of Chi was an external feeling or an internal feeling?

"From the outside," she declared. "From the outside. It was from the tornado that was going around."

Sam said that the experience sounded like that of a child at a circus, who just wanted to run around and spin.

"That's what I did," ruth responded. "That's what it felt like. And I spun around in one Direction, and then I spun around in the opposite direction."

"It sounds like you are very liberated," Sam said. "That you could do pretty much anything."

"Well, Dr. Mike taught us to let it move us," she responded. "He does what I call that 'healing dance', and so when I was standing, I just wanted to let it move me, and move me in whichever direction."

That's how I was taught, I said. When I was training, I never did any by rote Qi Gong exercises; rather, it was about the Qi entering you and working from inside to move you, as though directing your nervous system to move here and there, and entering your innate intelligence, which I consider the ultimate in Qi Gong…

Sam compared what ruth experienced to achieving a high level as an athlete.

"In sports," he began, "when someone gets to a certain level of athletic skills, it becomes effortless in our movements and capability to perform, and basically you're just dancing with the energy that the sport provides you, like as if you're coming down a mountain on skis, or if you're coming down a wave on a surfboard - it just flows. You're not just picking up a chess piece, but you're intentionally flowing with that chess piece and being able to really strike a blow."

I commented that muscle memory supposedly resides in a particular area of the brain, the basal ganglia, and you wonder if the highest experience in Qi Gong that I was describing, when the chi takes your body and move you, isn't acting at that part of the brain?

"Even in a chest move, I've always said that a chess player is a special type of athlete," Sam commented. "And after they figured out every option that a move can provide, they move with confidence, versus another person, who really doesn't know if he's falling into a trap. With a chess player, he picks up that piece and feels it in his hand, as though it's part of him, and you know it's strength, and it's capabilities, and you move it into a position of strength, and it's really an effortless move.

"And so, to me, that's what an athlete does. It doesn't matter if they're doing a bench press or a clean and jerk with barbells, it's the same feeling as if you're coming down a mountain, or coming down a wave.

"And so, with Qi Gong, when you become really confident with the chi, it's no longer a stranger, but a friend. And there's a difference. A lot of people treat it like a stranger, so they don't know what to make of it? 'Is it a dangerous stranger? Or is this a stranger who could be helpful to me? Will it become a friend of mine?'

"And after you do it, then you kind of eliminate all the risk, and you realize all the benefits, and then all of a sudden you start to flow with your friend. You walk in tandem with it down the road. Because it's your friend. And you have a common conversation with it..."

Then, I turned to Sam and asked how he was doing? He indicated that he was doing all right, so I invited others to share.

Whitney commented that she's been enjoying this conversation.

"I'm still holding onto the feeling that I had during the self-practice," she commented.

It happened that I was, too, so that I still had my eyes closed and was still feeling energy in my crown and chakra and higher third eye, and at those points above my ankles.

"But everything that's been said I relate to so much," she continued. "Where you either feel the external push to be moved or to move; where you feel that coming from within and the trust, like it's almost like a dance partner. That resonated very deeply in me and was very complementary to what I've been doing."

She talked about how it was that she was sitting in her bed in a semi-lotus position, so that she felt more grounded.

It happened that I was sitting that way, too, on Sam's couch, mostly because I couldn't stretch my legs out.

She commented that she hadn't done the self-practice in months and was worried that she wasn't going to perceive anything when she first started.

"But once I started, I was right back in it," she said.

She described how it was that she had the lights out, so that it was like she had a little altar for herself, and thanked me for offering this kind of virtual session.

I said that we would continue these sessions like this, and I didn't know why it was that I hadn't thought of it before, especially when so many from the study indicated that they weren't able to come for the sessions because it was too much to ask of them where they were having persistent long Covid symptoms and were still working, and the sessions were happening smack in the middle of the week.

"And we didn't know if it would work or not," Ruth asserted. "It worked when you were in Texas, but I kind of felt that it worked because there was the group of us there together to build energy together. But it worked with us all in different locations now, which surprises me…"

Ruth expressed her appreciation for Sam's insight and way of looking at Qi.

"For me, Qi Gong has involved a level of trust," she said. "Because it's very subtle, and you decide either, 'OK, I'm going to go with it', or 'I'm not.' Like a dance partner. Or flowing with the music. Or a run where everything is just in flow."

I shared about how it was that the exit interview study showed that those who did not have an experience of chi, did not improve with qi Gong for their long Covid symptoms. So, it seemed that an experience of chi was necessary to benefit from qi Gong.

"I think it's very easy to just dismiss it, because it's so subtle," ruth said. "It's not going to force itself on you. It's just there if you want it."

I definitely agreed and said that it was so foreign and unusual and out of the ordinary that it seems to me easy to dismiss; and to refer to it as "voodoo" and "primitive" and "backwards" and "unscientific" and "unusual" and "make believe" and not anything "based in reality."

"That's because it's not understood yet," Sam said. "When you understand something, then it becomes common knowledge."

Yes, I just wanted to make the point that to this day, I found it more surprising that people did perceive it and benefit from it, than not. I am not surprised that there were folks who could not perceive it, and I am not surprised that there were folks who did not benefit from it - For all the reasons I previously listed.

I shared that a participant (N.) from the first study cohort had related being greeted with significant skepticism from his coworkers when he shared about his Qi Gong experiences.

"They asked him what he was drinking," I said. "And then, when he told them he hadn't been drinking, they said, 'Well, then, what have you been smoking?"

So, I really appreciated that, for as different and as foreign as this approach was, so many people in the study (who were suffering from really serious problems related to long COVID) had availed and opened themselves to the possibility that there might be something to this Qi Gong approach and that it might help them.

"It's easier to tear something down than build something up," Sam declared. " Most people are lazy, so it's easier for them to just tear something down. People do that naturally…"

I asked my brother if he wanted to share?

My brother announced that he was in Costa Rica, and ruth expressed surprise, saying that she wouldn't expect it to work from so far away.

My brother said that he had a very intense experience, like he felt like he knew everyone in the group.

"The energy felt magnetic," he said. "The energy that was releasing out of the tips of my fingers, and I may have felt a little bit coming out of my forehead tonight, which I haven't felt in the past. I've been exposed to Qi Gong since 1990. I felt energy, but I haven't practiced it a lot."

He shared how inspiring it was to listen to the others.

"It is real," he declared, "and it does work. Regardless of wherever you may be, distance doesn't apply to this. There's a healing. Right now, my hands are still tingling at the tips, and my hands are still making a ball shape, like I'm folding clay."

He talked about our upbringing.

"Michael and I played a lot of tennis growing up," he said. "And I did a lot of sports, so I connected with Sam. And dancing; and it's so important to have that ability to dance, not only alone, but also with a partner, because, on the court, you want to be like Fred Astaire.

"And the muscle memory, yes, it does take time to create muscle memory, and that muscle memory gives you the confidence to go out and perform the sport that you love, or the dance that you love, with a degree of confidence, and also freedom, so you know your ability and what your level is; and you could tailor it if somebody is at a lower level; but if someone is at a higher level, it gives you some incentive to want to keep improving. In this opportunity, I'm so grateful to you guys for sharing it with me, because I have times that I do Qi Gong alone, but it's so great that there are actually people out there who participated in a study, one, so you should all feel very proud of yourselves to have taken on this challenge.

"Sure, people could say, 'What have you been drinking? What have you been smoking?' But for the people who experience this energy… Well, the universe is guiding us, right? So, it's out of our control. And I guess you do have to believe in it to feel it, but even if you don't believe in it, you can feel the magnetic pull."

"Tonight, I felt the magnetic pole," he continued. "Other times I felt heat, and that's when I'm working with someone else, maybe I feel the heat from their bodies. Of course, I've seen my brother do many forms of chi gong, but this one is so unique. Because the energy is coming from ourselves, and the forces are almost supernatural. And whether you're riding a wave, like Sam said, or you're playing chess - which is a great example, because Michael was a great chess player.

"I mean, Michael was great at everything. The weightlifting... Michael has a tremendous amount of experience beyond just being an amazing doctor and just human being. He's an amazing dancer. So when you bring up dance, it's connecting with him, and he knows that you're getting the chi. And it's basically corroborating the truth that it is happening, and it is working.

"I've never met any of you. I've never seen any of you. But yet I feel like I know you. Like I listen to each one's voice, and I could tell who is speaking. And I feel like we're all in the same room almost.

"Because I don't know about you all, but a lot of times I have my eyes closed, and you could almost like visualize certain things. And each one of you brought your descriptions of what happened tonight, and what happened other nights, like when Mike was in Texas, and there were things that started to trigger, and I still feel the energy in my hands. When we were kids, we used to play with magnets a lot. So, it's like you feel the energy of attraction with the magnets clicking together. But then, you can turn the magnets the other way and you feel that energy of repulsion and the magnets wanting to come apart.

"Yeah, there are those people out there who are working, and their time is consumed with making sure their rent is paid, and their bills are paid, and their car has gas, and there different appointments and what not. But as we sit here, it's like, yes, you have to be in a place of presence and peacefulness that, like one of you said, was by your bed, and in darkness, and you were comfortable.

"And you were worried, 'Oh, I haven't done this in a while', but you did it tonight, and you don't have to do it on a regular basis. It's nice to, of course. But everyone has their lives to live, and it's just really gratifying that you gave yourself the patience and the time to say, 'OK, maybe it will work. I'm willing.' And it did. And it signifies some kind of meaning and purpose behind this..."

Then, Sam finally volunteered his experience.

"I think it's important for me to share," he began, "because I imagine everyone will become like me at a stage when you get so close I guess to the end and things start to fail in your body.

"Of course, the key thing failing in my body is my lungs. So, when I was standing, and my arms began to pull apart, they went up to shoulder height, which I believe was just representing my lungs or my chest cavity where my hands were, because it felt like my hands were reflecting the energy from my chest.

"But every breath felt really good. And my arms stayed up effortlessly. I could have held my arms up like this forever at that level with what it felt like with my arms outstretched at shoulder level. And every breath kept keeping them up. Every inhalation and exhalation of my breath. And it felt really, really good.

"So, I felt strong. And then, of course, it wore down after a while, and my arms did become heavier and started to slowly go down.

"And when my arms came down to my sides… Well, let me go back a little bit. I have these tremors in my right hand ever since I got my problem with my chest. And Mike says it looks like early-stage Parkinson's. But I don't think it's Parkinson's. It could be, but I think there's a little bit more that's accelerating it. Because when my hands went down, my right hand really started to shake. It shook uncontrollably. And I was going to try to stop it, but then I said, 'You know what? I'll just let it shake.' And so it just started to shake really hard, and then it stopped all of a sudden.

"And so, what I think is happening is that when my hands were at shoulder level, and my chest was breathing effortlessly and my hands were being suspended up there, I think it gave me a chance to feel how the chest should feel like when it's healthy. Because every breath of mine is work for me now. And during the practice, it wasn't work. It was actually feeling very good. Every breath felt like I could actually breathe normally?

"Anyway, when my hands came down, my right hand and my left hand started to shake. And my right hand shook really violently. And then it stopped. And I think if I was to try to speculate what might be happening, and I have no scientific basis to really say, and this is just sort of what my mind thinks, is that the bad energy in my lungs was exiting my fingers and going towards the ground, dissipating, and that's what the shaking was… It was the bad energy flowing out of my fingers.

"Now, it kind of sounds kind of funny, it sounds like something out of marvel cartoon characters, but the thing is, that's what it felt like, because all of the sudden, it stopped, and my hands were very calm and relaxed, and I felt very relaxed.

"However, my breathing was a little heavier. Not as heavy as it usually is. So, I felt like it helped me a little bit with my breathing.

"So, this exercise was really good at maybe getting my parasympathetic nervous system involved in calming me down to a point where I was able to relax a bit more.

"Because, like I said, every breath is work. And that work engages my sympathetic nervous system, and then I go into this fight or flight scenario, and it affects my whole body: Digestive system - My hormonal system - My immune system - And everything else.

"Because when you're in a fighting mode, a lot of these things are either enhanced and releasing a lot of adrenaline and corticosteroids, in case you get hurt, because then it fights and heal you quickly; but if you get too much of it, it causes stressful things to happen and degradation to occur.

"So, for a short time, it's very good. But when the sympathetic nervous system is engaged 24-seven, then you are really in a very terrible state.

"So, this chi gong got me into a more parasympathetic nervous system state, allowing me to deal with my bad situation in my body.

"And I only say this and tell you this because everyone is going to reach a certain level of my stage towards the end. Because I've just been with too many people who have passed away, and everybody goes through the stages, like Kubler-Ross five stages of mourning and all that.

"So, this is one of these things that we will all go through, and maybe chi gong will help you get through the tough moments and give everyone a little peace. Because every little thing that's good is very significant when you're at a stage like this."

As he concluded, I reminded the group of Whitney's quote: "Any amount of better is better..."

CHAPTER FIFTEEN

Sunday, July 6, 2025

I told Sam that I'd visited with Bubbles and helped her with her problem of cervical radiculopathy; however, I was afraid that her concern for Sara was such that she wasn't going to take my help again.

"I think you can only do so much for an old friend," Sam said. "Anyway, there are a lot more far worse things that can happen to you. I think you can only do so much. That's really good that you're concerned about a friend. Now, you can just wait until she needs you.

Sam asked what I had planned for work in the coming week. I said I had the week off to assist my father, but I didn't think that I was going to go to Carson City, because Bubbles was in town through Wednesday, and I didn't think I could leave here where she might be in need of my assistance.

Then, after Bubbles leaves, I said I was more worried about him than my father.

"Oh, that's OK," he said. "I think your attention should definitely be on your father than me. I would think that that would bother me a lot. But then, when you're in it that deep, does it really bother you? Unless it really frustrates you, so maybe he recognizes that he forgets and gets really upset about it, feeling like, 'I can't think and do things like the way I used to.'"

"I guess the frustration is worse than the not knowing, "he concluded. "It's kind of interesting that you go through life, and you tell people something that's truthful, you expect people to believe you and to go along with you, because you've been the leader, and your word has been something that people have followed. But then, all of a

sudden, you don't have that level of respect for what you do and you say… That must be very, very frustrating. It will seem like you're a 'nobody."

Exactly, and here my father had previously been a "Captain industry."

"That must be very frustrating," Sam continued. "It's like a leader who loses his edge in battle, because he's not thinking correctly, and causes his soldiers to commit suicidal acts because he's just not reasoning properly, but he doesn't want to give up his command.

"And then you have to stand up to that leader. Do you say, 'No, you're thinking is totally wrong'? Or do you have to go along with them?

"And then, do you force it on them? Or do you do it later?"

"It's pretty tough," he concluded. "I'm sure I'll be getting to that situation, as well."

I wasn't - I didn't think Sam had much longer to live.

"I hope I'm more understanding," he said. "You know, May has been telling me that there have been a lot more flash floods in Texas, and a lot of people are missing or have been killed. And how does one die in a flash flood? Either your battered to death or you drown. And I keep thinking, 'Drowning in a flash flood and not being able to breathe… That's eventually how I'm going to get. I'm not going to be able to breathe.' But I'm very fortunate, because my decrease in breathing is coming gradually. So, I've been practicing my lack of breathing all of this time.

"Because I've gone through so many iterations of not breathing, from choking, to drowning on just a little bit of water in my throat, due to the lack of air when I do too much activity. So, I've been preparing myself for that final moment where I don't have air. Whereas these people drowning in a flash flood, it was instant. They never had any practice. This was it. They were drowning. And you're not going to come out of it. And how frightening that could be.

"But, then again, since I had my drowning experience, I know how frightening that can be, but at the very, very end, it's very relaxing.

"And so I can imagine that for those people, it was very, very frightening until the very end, when their mind puts them at ease."

Yes, the freeze response.

"So, I could imagine what they went through, versus for me - I get to know, practice and practice and practice. It's sort of like, 'Death by 1000 cuts.' Each cut gets me closer to it. And a computer program trying to analyze a situation, and playing all the different

scenarios, and saying, 'Oops, no, this is when I died. Let's try another scenario.... Oops, well, that is when I died', so you keep doing all of these different scenarios, and then you realize, 'I'm not going to find a scenario that I come back alive.' So it's a really interesting situation I am in.

"And I think it's really fortunate that I get this opportunity to have that. Because I've always wanted to study things really well, and even in my final study here, I get to study and analyze. And since all the scenarios end up with the same conclusion, it makes it sort of interesting - The end result is always the same.

"So, I'm thinking about all these poor people who didn't have a chance to witness other things. They just only had this one opportunity to experience drowning - though I don't wish what I'm going through on anyone. But since it has to happen, I'm sort of happy that it's happening this way for me..."

Before the External Qi Gong treatment, Sam shared that the week-long evaluations at Stanford had really set him back physically, so that he had not recovered, and ultimately felt that they had done him in injustice.

With Sam lying on the massage table, I connected with him energetically the moment I extended my hand towards the left side of his body as he was lying there. It took me in a circle around him, moving down his left arm, to his legs, up around his right arm, until I felt my left hand become filled with energy, for chi emission, such that it went to his crown chakra area.

I told him that I had never had an experience like that. I didn't tell him that it left me feeling rather odd, because there I was sending energy to a place that I only associated with receiving divine energy from the universe?

This was an area of the body that I just didn't mess with when it came to bioenergy. I never scan someone's crown chakra. That's an area of the body that I consider sacrosanct and not to be interacted with. Originally, I'd been taught this was where a person connected with the Universal Qi; now, it was becoming more akin to connecting with the "divine" and "Mother Spirit", etc. Hence, it was becoming even less possible for me to imagine Qi emission happening there!

At the same time, my crown chakra was becoming quite activated.

In retrospect, I wondered if I was serving us a conduit for the universal chi?

I asked if he was experiencing anything?

"Just a calmness," he replied, weekly. "I feel more relaxed. My chest is not as armed and compensating."

My left hand continued to stay at his crown chakra emitting energy.

Earlier, before dinner, Sam talked about how it was that he felt that he was degrading and deteriorating, getting weaker and less functional every day. Every day, he said that something that he could do from the day before, he could no longer do the next day, so that it was watching this degradation, and he didn't know how long he could continue, especially because he felt so useless and incapable of offering assistance. He described not being able to do the dishes or make the bed. He offered a lot of metaphors that I can't remember now. Like that he was being pulled down by the water and couldn't surface anymore. He was drowning, and he couldn't push back against the current - The flow of the river was too powerful for him.

Meanwhile, the energy took me on repeated games of "twister", putting my left arm in an arm lock as following the energy twisted my body around.

"And I have no idea why?" I said.

It felt like the energy was interacting with my lower chakras, and then to my left hip, where I suffer from a kind of weakness there from putting pressure there.

Hence, it would make sense that I would need and receive healing there…

The energy left my hand, but stayed at my lower chakra and crown chakra.

I sat on the couch and told Sam that this is not taken anywhere near as long as I was expecting. It was 7:11, so there was lots of time before the group practice at 7:30.

Sam thanked me for what I'd done.

With Sara and May talking in the background, Sam got up from the massage table and I went about folding it back up and putting it back into its place.

Sam asked me what my focus had been?

I said that I just went into it doing the usual, without any preconceived ideas.

And then I shared how surprised I was that I would be sending healing energy to his crown chakra?

"I'm sure there was a need for that," he responded.

I didn't ask him to elaborate.

Sam indicated that he was going to lie down on the couch. He said that he was not as short of breath as he was before.

"It usually feels like I'm in a constant vice in my chest," he said. "Anyway, it was good.

"It's funny: If I have a good night's sleep, there's a time that I wake up, sometimes at 1 o'clock in the morning, sometimes it's three or four, and I feel normal. I feel good. I can move my arms. It feels good.

"But it only lasts for a short while. And doing that period I feel like, 'Oh man, there's hope! And if I can just keep this going…"

"But I know, in the back of my head, it's going to dissipate and disappear in a matter of minutes, and I won't feel this normality, and I'm back to where I am right now, with my chest clamped.

"I feel like there's this energy buzzing through me, and it's not a good energy - Instead of bees, it's like hornets, buzzing through me. It's interesting. Very interesting, Mike…"

Sam excused himself. As I sat waiting, I pondered Sam's condition. It would seem to me that it was an auto-immune system that was the source of the scarring. Immunosuppressants weren't offered, because studies had shown that they were not effective.

But I still wanted to think that there was hope now, being that potential sources of scarring that his body was reacting against were no longer a source of exposure and getting into a system: he wasn't being exposed to the silicon spray or the carpet fibers with his ski school and endless slope; the house had been rid of asbestos. Those things have been taken away. Hence, it seemed that there weren't those sources of fibrosis anymore. If that were the case, then why wouldn't the scarring be arrested? Why would Sam's condition worsen? Wasn't it possible that it would be stabilized? Put his condition on hold?

Sam returned.

"It's interesting," he began and coughed heavily. "That whole thing where I wake up at night and feel normal for a short while… It's a really neat feeling. Because it's that same feeling when I'm at the verge of being able to accomplish something that I've been working on.

"But the thing is, in reality, I lose it. I lose those accomplishments. And it drives you hopeless. You just feel hopeless. It's like someone teasing you: 'Here, you can have this… Nope… Taking it away from you.… Here, you can have it again… Nope, you can't have it.…' For my psyche, it's just a matter of, how long am I able to live with that? There's going to be a point where I just say, 'You know, there is no hope. Except for one. And that is, to eliminate this completely by not existing."

"Right now, I know I have that card, and to me, that's a winning card," he continued. "To just say, 'You're never going to get it, and I can't handle being in this state of never having hope."

"So, my game plan is to not exist," he concluded. "And not be without hope.

"And I know that day is going to come; and that is the best option, because there is no other option.

"So, I am wondering, How long can I survive without Hope? That's what it's going to come down to.

"Because right now I'm living in a state where I'm struggling all the time. And being without hope is a state that one can survive in for a long, long while. And it will be interesting when I start getting to that point and see how long I can survive that way?"

My phone rang. It was my brother.

"Is it time, Mike?" Sam asked.

I said it was 7:26 PM.

"It's time," Sam responded…

I answered my brother's call, but asked him to give us a minute, as Sam and I were having a serious conversation.

Then, turning to Sam, I declared that none of us was going to live forever, and tried to convey that he wasn't alone, and we were all essentially in the same place he was.

"Sure," he responded, "but when you're thinking about it that way, you're thinking that if you did that forever, you'd be living with your same quality of life. I mean, do you think of yourself living forever with your skin coming off, and not being able to walk? No, nobody thinks about that. When people think about immortality, they're thinking about something like a vampire, that still looks pretty good, can dance, can sing. But that's not realistic.

"So, yeah, no one lives forever, but the thing is, what state will you be in? What is your physical state? What is your mental state as you're approaching that end point?

"And you're not going to be perfect till the very end. Not even close.

"I can't walk. I can't do the dishes. I can't even sign bills. All I am is becoming a sponge that's taking things, because that's what it's going to take to keep me alive. I'm requiring all of this support and taking from other people's lives.

"If I were able to be functional and to add a certain low level of being able to help out, do the dishes, make my bed… Well, then that's worth living. Because I'm still contributing. But when I stop contributing, that's a different story. Then, I can't be useful anymore.

No one wants to be dragging around a body that's totally useless, and saying, 'Here, meet my friend, Sam. He can't get up, but he's here with us. Maybe we can have him prop open the door.' You know, there's a point where I become totally useless, and I have to figure out where that point is? And the problem with my situation right now is my degradation is occurring quickly enough that I see its progression, and I wonder, 'Is it tomorrow that I won't be able to get up? I'm going to get worse tomorrow, but I'm still going to be able to stand up. But instead of being able to walk to the kitchen, I won't be able to walk that far.... I'll only be able to walk to the door.' So, when is it that one says, 'At this point, things should be sort of stopped'?"

He said that he'd had to see his dentist, Dr. Kubota, earlier in the day.

"He found two cavities," he said. "He fixed one cavity, and tomorrow he's going to fix a major one that's underneath a cap. And I'm thinking, 'It really doesn't pain me that much. Is it worth the fix?'"

"The other thing is my business license," he continued. "It's due. But I'm not running my business now. I can't. But I still submitted my business permit for the next year, just in case I feel better. Maybe they'll be a turnaround? Maybe I'll start to improve?"

"So, it's not like I'm giving up hope," he concluded. "I'm still doing everything that I can for a future…"

Listening, I knew Sam was right.

The other day with Sara in Monterey (after leaving Bubbles), some shells got in between my sandals and bare feet and left me to bleed with some cuts and scrapes. But the wounds were getting better with time.

I get injured, and I just get better, I thought. His lungs have been injured, but they are not recovering. They are not healing. That's the difference between me and him. He is not undergoing healing. He is just undergoing more wounding and developing deeper wounds. His "wounds" are not getting better. They're just getting worse, and he's sliding closer and closer to death.

I bowed my head.

Don't I understand how terrible this is for him? I thought. How overwhelming and fear inspiring this is? How could I be asking so much of him?...

I turned to the other folks on the call. Ruth and Whitney had shown up for the virtual Qi Gong self-practice, so we decided to begin, and I initiate the self-practice.

I was feeling energy in an interesting way, such that more than a breeze, it was more like particulates present against my hands. And it was everywhere against my hands. And the energy was drawing my hands closer than usual, like two or 3 inches apart, rather than the usual 6 to 8 inches apart.

Ultimately, I did feel my hands being spread apart in the usual arcing fashion. However, as my hands were on my lap, I still had the feeling that I was holding a very distinct energy ball that was encompassing every aspect of my hands.

My hands were then directed upwards by the energy, and following it by just bending at my elbows , until there was the activation of my crown chakra at about my hands, reaching shoulder level.

But then my hands were directed even higher than my shoulder level, and rather than just palms up, my palms were facing my shoulders.

And the reason for all these differences, I did not know?

My hands were directed downward to my lap again, and I just sat with the energy.

I shared with the others how it was that there are lots of points in the hands that are associated with the heart chakra and the heart in general when it comes to the acupuncture, meridians and acupuncture points.

Perhaps you have heart and head practice? I always thought that the activation of the crown chakra was key, but perhaps the connection with the Universal Qi at the hands was just as important? Maybe you could fuse your heart and head this? I know that my worst regrets in life or biggest questions in life were when I put my head above my heart, or vice versa.

My hands became directed with energy towards my heart chakra and then sending energy outwards. And then the pattern continued, back-and-forth, energy towards my heart, and then sending energy out and away from my heart.

Again, I didn't know why? Perhaps I should talk with Qi Gong masters to see what they think, but, really, I didn't think they (or anyone) had a "direct line to the truth" when it came to this unchartered science called Energy Medicine.

There was energy, particularly in my first three fingers, and it seemed that there was this alignment with my mid sternum. And it made sense, because these were ribs that were most concave and closed up in my chest.

I thought about Bubbles and her telling me that I keep myself closed from others.

"Because you thought no one could hold a candle to me," she'd said.

It struck me that essentially all of us had chest issues: I held my stress in my chest; Sam had his interstitial lung disease; ruth had her atrial fibrillation and palpitations.

I was feeling a prominence of energy at my third eye, and my head was directed downwards.

Finally, my hands were directed to hang downwards from my shoulders, and at this point, I invited others to share.

Ruth commented that this was the first time she'd seen Sam and said that there was a light shining from his left side and asked him to turn his body, so to determine if it might be the light coming from the window or an aura?

"Nope, it's not from the window," she said. "I had first saw a shadow from Sam's chest, more on the left side than the right side, and then I saw a light come up from his chest on the left side that has moved to the center of his chest now."

"Well, my left side is worse," Sam responded. "It's only 30% functional, where is my right is 45 to 50% functional. So, there is a difference between the left lung and the right."

"It seems there were a lot of things in my hands," he continued. "My hands felt very heavy, not by weight, but by weight of energy, I guess. They didn't feel like they were a massively heavy; it just felt like there was something in there, like energy or whatever, and it was just a lot more concentrated in my hands - And it still is…"

My brother indicated that there was a lot going on for him.

"I feel the energy in my hands," he began. "I was feeling the ball of energy, and then I opened my hands up to the sky and my finger we're tingling and still are. And I can feel some source… Some healing source… And I can't explain it…"

He commented about with ruth said about seeing the light come out of Sam.

"There's a connection there. And of course we're all praying for Sam. He's got something, but that doesn't mean he can't recover from it. And she's seeing something that is very important.

"And I don't want Sam to think that things are over yet. Far from over right now. However, bad it is. This woman is seeing something that's a light source of energy that's working some healing that's unexplainable, but we are are all coming together on this Wednesday night in a comfortable zone and chills and healing is going through our bodies, and we're seeing things that could be the light from the

window, but when you look at it both ways, is coming from something else that you can't explain.

My brother talked about the experience of jumping into the ocean with his surfing gear, aligning with Sam's experience, surfing and in sports in general and then commenting about the place that he was in and how Sam talked about how it was that we would all get to that place sooner or later.

"And you're in a tough spot right now, but remember, the comeback is always better than the setback. For whatever you might think of. We're all just here temporarily. Your soul is super genuine, and you've got to experience a lot of great things in life. But it's not over yet. Michael's there. And there's what ruth observed. That sparkling light."

"And you're the foundation on which everything is going to grow, in terms of figuring out how to get somebody to a constant state of chi gone? So, there's a reason and a purpose for everything.

"These are really special times and it's amazing that we can sit down and Michael say, 'OK, let's get started, put your hands out', and start feeling the synergy. What if we could do that all day long? Maybe Michael is going to find a way to make that a reality? I think he will. If anyone can, he can."

"It's not how you start, it's how you finish," my brother declared. "We all want to be honest, humble, dedicated, trustworthy, fair. We all want to be the dance partner that someone would want. The partner. We're all trying to grow. Michael's gonna go on to discover ways to do that with Qi Gong and so are we.

"Michael is just a conduit for all of this energy that's already flowing in the universe. He's guiding us because he's a master of this. He's a master of many things, but this is his passion in life.

"So, those are the things that I'm feeling. It leaves me with a lot of humility, like it all almost brings me to my knees. Because you've gotta be knocked down to your knees sometime to find the essence of good within yourself and the other people around you.

"So, this is not the beginning of something great, because this has been going on for thousands of years. It could be from the beginning of time?"

"This energy stuff let me tap into my abilities and see things like I've never seen before and put myself into places. I never thought that I would get to a point where I could share things like this with people like you all, and my brother. Over the last month, I've been finding that I'm more kind, and more gracious, and more confident, and more concerned about people and being willing to give them my

prize possessions, like tennis rackets, and paddle boards and trophies. Because they're just things, and can all be replaced. But people's energies and feelings and positive thoughts. And ruth is tapping into something, and I think you should go with ruth in terms of the light. And Mike is going to continue this.

"And there might just be a few of us on the phone today, but I can see this really going big, and it will change all of your all lives in a significant and humbling way."

Just then, my brother announced that his crown chakra had become activated.

"I felt it," he said. "It's like, 'Hey, what happened?', and they'll be a time when this is the way that people's trauma gets healed. And diagnosed. Not by robots and AI and computers. Yes, they're fabulous things because they run numbers and they're important to quantify and offer a qualitative type of analysis that we all rely on.

"So, these things will work in conjunction, but it will really be Qi Gong That is the higher source and look to a higher light to do this.

"Time will tell, obviously, but you all know, because if not, you wouldn't come back on a Wednesday night for this."

My brother commented about our lives, and how it was that we had to do everything together.

"We each have our gifts. Michael is really good at getting us to this point, and then, what does he do? He asked for feedback?"

"You should really be proud of yourselves, and you're embarking on something that can change many types of things if we can continue to do this. We should be doing this in these really huge places. Everywhere we should be doing this. Not just when you're sick. We're feeling bad, no, but all the time. All the time. Like constant. Just like breathing. You don't think about breathing. You take it for granted. But you can hear now that it's difficult for Sam to breathe. And like he said, maybe all of us are going to be like that one day. And I know that we have lung cancer in our family. We have heart disease."

My brother commented that he wondered what was Sam's age? I tried to relate that it was Sam's birthday next week and tried to steer him to finish his sharing.

"Yeah, I'm done, but Sam is not," he continued. "You're far from it. My brother is going to do everything that he can to help you. We are, too. All of us in this room. And more people that don't even know are going to. And now you have to start believing. Your life has been a good one. It's not why does this happen to good people, it's, 'Maybe this is the experiment that michael has been waiting for?'

And this is the time to really show the world that this is not just something to be taken lightly.

"People say, 'What are you talking about? Have you been drinking? Have you been smoking something?' No, this is something they're going to say, 'Wow, this works. And here's proof.'

"He's got proof all up and down the board about how he's been able to help people. Why can't he help in this situation, too?

"So, I'm just saying from me to you, Sam, just stay positive. Talk to yourself with as much positivity as you can. Because that will help start this constant flow of bioenergy. The Qi Gong - That Mike can't explain the why's and how's. We're all with you in this thing.

"In any event, don't give up. We really care. And Mike really cares. Sam is a big part of his healing journey. Why do you think we're having it in this fashion? Healing Sam?

"And Sam, I'm sure you have doctors coming and going all the time. But then you have Michael. That's the one.

"And I'm not biased. in 1993, I saw it. I don't know how it happened. But it happened. I can't just put it out of my mind..."

"Definitely, there are moments where things felt like they were normal," Sam responded, thoughtfully. "The way it was when I never thought about breathing and just went about my business. And now it's always on my mind, and when it's on your mind, it becomes work.

"So, there are moments with Qi Gong that you don't think about breathing. You just naturally do it. And when you get into that state, things feel a lot more normal.

"And, so, yeah, I think there is a strong mental aspect, as well as a Qi Gong state – which has a lot to do with mental state.

"The nice thing about Qi Gong is that you have both mental and physical, because you can feel it through your body, and it's just connecting all the dots within your body to work in harmony. And when it works in harmony, then you get to a more relaxed state, allowing everything to be more neutral. And when it's all neutral, it starts to function as it should. And I think that's how our bodies evolutionarily have been developed to function, without having to think.

"You shouldn't have to think about breathing when you're at Macy's, looking for merchandise. It should be all automatic: your ability to walk; your ability to balance; your ability to see, hear, speak; to have all of your senses come alive; and it's all done automatically. So, yeah, it's a good feeling when they do that.

"However, when something goes awry with a system, then there's an emphasis on that, and it can throw you all off balance. So, it's nice that Qi Gong can put you into a balance.

"But I don't think it's a permanent balance. However, with practice, you can make it last longer and longer and longer.

"And there is a point of stability where you can function more freely, and that's what we need to get to. But it all depends on your disease state. How bad it is, and how it dominates? Because you can't always put things aside when something is wrong.

"It's like trying to ignore a flat tire while you're driving down the freeway; maybe you can stop and put some air in it and then try for a short while? But the air eventually goes out. So, until the tire is completely repaired and may be replaced, you're just doing a Band-Aid effect.

"I think this is very good and it has made me feel a lot better, and I hope it allows me to carry on a little bit further, in a more peaceful state…"

Looking on the monitor, the others who'd joined us had left, and I indicated that we were calling it a night.

"Hang in there, Sam," my brother added. "I'll catch a wave for you. And I know you'll catch another one, too. Like, you're with me in spirit. I live in the best place in Costa Rica for waves and surfing, and today something drew me out there. Think positive."

"Your brother is a brilliant person," Sam conceded. "He's like a beautiful mind. He sees connections and everything. I have a bit of that, too. It makes us see the world as a matrix, rather than individual things. It's really good that he does this. He just needs to hone it."

I apologized, saying I let my brother go on because last week I felt he'd projected an energy that was helpful.

"Well, the sun projects energy, too," Sam said. "And it's everywhere. The thing is, we make sunlight into solar power by concentrating it and directing it properly. Otherwise, you just have a lot of radiant heat."

"Call it my imagination," I said, "but I did think he sent healing energy last week."

"But in a group session, you can't have a singular person talk for that long," Sam declared, disgusted. "You lose people."

"He's a genuine person," Sam continued. "He is on the right track. He's able to see things and connect things. He just needs to practice how to categorize better in his mind."

And maybe take some criticism, I added.

"Yeah, well, I don't think he likes outside criticism," Sam commented. "He has to find a criticism within himself. Maybe listening to himself on a tape?

"Because he's intelligent. He knows what a good speaker sounds like. He's been listening to good speakers all his life. So that he thinks in his mind that he's one of the good speakers, because these good speakers are capable of taking all sorts of things and bringing them down into a concise comment. And able to eliminate things that take away from that.

"So, he just needs to clean it up. I mean, he has the start of a genius. I think it runs in your family. The thing is, he just needs to learn how to control his genius. Because if you don't hone it in, then you start to drift. And when you drift, you're not as constructive as you could've been.

"It's no fault of his. He just needs to practice. Just like an athlete who has all of this ability. He has the right body proportions, the right muscle strength. But he doesn't know how to be disciplined. And for that reason, he keeps losing. He gets close to the top, but he never makes it.

"Anyway, I enjoy your brother and his character," Sam concluded, "but I feel sad for the other people in your group."

I told Sam that I had let my brother intentionally go on because of the benefits that Sam had received during the last Qi Gong self-practice. Unlike any other Qi Gong self-practices, he had had the most significant response in that one, both in his breathing and for his tremor last week, and it seemed to me that the ingredient that was present then that had not been present in any other session was my brother. As a result, I was willing to let him go on and on to put forward that kind of energy.

"No," Sam asserted. "It was you. I was only listening to you. Because you were leading it. It didn't have anything to do with the other people. You may think that by having many people, it makes a difference, but it's about how deep the individual dwells into it. And I've been dwelling into it with you for a long time.

"Like I said, I trust you. I wouldn't feel as comfortable with other Qi Gong masters. Because there's a disconnect. I don't know them. You, I know very, very well. And so, I know where you're coming from. There's no questioning when you say something. Or if I do question it, it's because this is something new, and you haven't brought it up before, or something like that, or just didn't fit with who you are. But that's rare, rare. It doesn't happen."

Sara wondered if my relationship with my brother didn't have an effect on me?

"If his energy wasn't especially potent on you?" she asked.

"I think you've been ignoring your brother a lot in the past," Sam asserted. "And this is the first time you feel there is a strong bond between you two. And that you don't want to lose that bond. Because when you were dealing with your mom, there was a friction between you and your brother. Tremendous friction, actually.

"And you could say that it was the situation with the house, and it was a situation from your childhood. And it was neat when you made peace with him, and you started to feel like things were working. So, the passing of your mom really brought you two together.

"And I don't think you want to lose that. Because it was the first time you really felt like, 'I have a good brother.' Or, 'I have a brother.' And you don't want to lose family.

"That's my feeling. I could be totally wrong."

No, he was completely mostly correct. Except that immediate family had always been really relatively dangerous to me, except for my grandfather.

"So, it's up to you," Sam continued. "It's just a feeling that I got.

"But I can see now that you and him… Well, he has a great respect for you. He talks about you more than he talks about me. There was the whole section about how he imagines you run your office; and what you wear, how you deal with your patients. How your work with Qi Gong has really influenced him now.

"And he admires what you're doing, and if I were you, I wouldn't want to lose that by saying something stupid.

"So, it's sad that your mom passed away, and there was a lot of friction with the house and the way she was being taken care of, and to be honest with you, the little you told me about your nephew, his son - It's like they were both kind of taking advantage of your mom."

Sam began to cough.

"I'm coughing because I'm really not 100% sure of that point," he said. "It's just a feeling I got."

Interesting that lack of certainty would lead to worsening of his symptoms? I thought. Because he was certainly right about one thing: He didn't have to question himself. Perhaps that was part of what was killing him? As I always said of him, he was literally humble to a fault!

"It seems like you're seeing a good deal of satisfaction with the way that things are turning out, and maybe he didn't have a lot of respect for his son, either. But now he has tremendous respect for his son, just like he has tremendous respect for you."

Maybe it went even further than that, and my father didn't have a lot of respect for me, and now he does?

And it might be the same way with my stepmother? And I could embrace that?

"So, it was nice for you to let him go on, though maybe not for the other participants," Sam continued. "But, for you, you were like the best psychiatrist he could possibly have... By letting him go on.

"I think from this point on, you're going to get closer with family."

"I think you're very fortunate to have a family," he concluded. "It's never too late…"

It was 9 o'clock, and I suggested we let Sam get some rest, though I asked if we should do the evening Qi Gong exercise with Lee Holden together?

Sam answered in the affirmative, though later sara would tell me that she thought this was a mistake, and that I was pushing Sam too hard…

Just before leaving, Sam commented about his Pulmonology Rehab appointment early that day, in which he underwent another six-minute diagnostic oxygen test.

"The respiratory therapist commented, 'You did very well. You had a good pace. You made it'," he said. "But I've never felt this bad doing a six-minute walk before. I'd like to appreciate his encouragement, but what does that encouragement mean? Does it mean, 'Oh, we have hope for you. You're going to get better'? I doubt that. Where I have been slipping down this far, all of a sudden, I'm going to make a U-turn? I don't think so. I'm always anxious to see what my options are. Maybe tomorrow I'll wake up and I'll feel super good? And I'll be able to do this and that and think, 'Oh, man, that was a lot easier than the day before.' But so far I haven't found that day."

Sam thanked me for the yesterday's Qi Gong treatment and self-practice.

"Also, it was interesting, where ruth thought she saw an aura around me," he commented. "I've always had an around me. People have always said that. Ever since I was a little kid. So, it didn't surprise me, because people who are into these things have told me, 'Oh, you have a big aura.' I've always been told that."

"I don't believe it, though," he added. "I don't know what it means. Is it that you need to get glasses?"

Sara commented that ruth was able to see energy with her eyes.

"When Mike would go and treat someone," she added, "Ruth would move so that she would have a line of sight to be able to see it."

"Well, you know, impressionists see the world differently than the artist before them, "Sam said. "The artist before them saw really sharp lines of distinction, and the impressionist saw shades. Who knows what someone sees and what it means?"

We didn't have the technology to know yet, I contended.

With that, Sam thanked us, and we were on our way...

CHAPTER SIXTEEN

Sunday, July 13, 2025

Sam commented that, in the future, he wanted to do the Qi Gong session virtually and not from his home.

"I feel like everybody's thinking about me, instead of thinking about themselves," he said. "So, I would rather eliminate myself out of that picture, because there's a little bit more anxiety on my part. In fact, I'm having these dreams that I'm taking care of people with all of these strange issues, and so it's just making me feel uncomfortable."

He also offered some thoughts regarding my brother.

"I'm not as tolerant as I was, so I need to focus on concise things," he said. "Your brother means well, but I don't think I can listen to him discuss things anymore, unless it's very concise and to the point."

"Nothing against him," he added. "Everybody pictures the world around them a certain way, and some people create the world very strongly and want things just the way they want them. It's like when I was young, I used to play with all kinds of army soldiers that look like little statues figures that look like little soldier men. For instance, I had a World War II set, where one guys throwing a hand grenade, and another is talking on a walkie-talkie, and another has a bazooka, and another one is standing at attention, and another has a rifle with a bayonet on it. And each person is very specific, and they have a role. So, you play this army with this world of yours, and each person has a certain role and character and personality that you create. And you create this image and this world. And your brother reminds me of people that I know who created their own world around them. They expect people to be a certain way, and as you know, if I did that to you and expected you to be a certain way all the time, you would not be very free to grow.

"And a lot of people expect others to be a certain way, and if they act differently, then they grow out of favor very easily, and don't allow people to grow and change and become different people. It's because they're very rigid. So, they build a world around them with people who they paint a certain way, and when these people change, like the guy with the bazooka, and he doesn't fire the bazooka anymore, and is now a rifleman, or a person standing at attention… Well, then they kind of discard that person, because you always want him to be a bazooka guy and always counted on him shooting the bazooka. So, now you just tossed that person out, and I feel some people are like that… That if you change in any way, then you're out of the world, and they don't like you as they used to, because they always expect you to be a certain way.

"And when your brother was talking, and certainly, he already has a picture of who you are and what you should be and things like that, I keep getting the feeling that if you change a little bit, then you'll grow out a favor with him. I felt that when you were describing him when I didn't even know him at all, and you were out of his favor when he envisioned you a certain way. Now, he envisions you in a different way, which is acceptable in his world. So, now he praises you, and I hear that quite a bit. And I wonder, 'What has made him change that way?'

"What I'm trying to say here is that I think some people are more fragile than others, and it's hard to be a certain image for people, so that if I change, I know that I go out a favor with them very easily.

"And it's difficult, because I go, 'Well, should I maintain a certain image for them? Or can I just be myself and change and be very Protean in my shape and my character?'

"Maybe that's just me, but throughout my life that's how I've dealt with people.

"I find that, for you, you're a very open person and you accept people, although you have your limits…"

Sam indicated he had to get off the phone to help May. To my surprise, though, Sam called back. His birthday was next week, and I told him that if he wanted, I would bring over some food from Ikeda's, and even drive him to the skating rink to visit with friends there, and then, to the Vietnamese restaurant just down the road to celebrate with those folks?

"May is taking me out for dinner," he responded, "and I don't want to be rushing anything and putting her into my schedule.... You're trying to do a wonderful thing for me, and I appreciate it, but it can create a conflict.

"I appreciate everything you've done. I've really enjoyed your friendship, and I was very fortunate that we ran into each other at the Rink and made the friendship that we've had.

"And like I said, you have a very accepting personality, and you accept more things than most people. But we all have our limits, don't we?"

He laughed.

"I always think about your friend who was African-American... Ben... And he was a pretty cool guy, but you got upset with him, and I just remember how you just really admired him, and I felt very sorry when things went south with you two."

Yes, I should have been more tolerant when he shared that antisemitic stuff.

"Well, I don't think it was right of him, and I just felt bad for him because you did so much for him and your friendship," he replied. "I don't think you have to regret anything. It was how you felt at the time. And your actions were just very appropriate at the time, because you have a stake in that.

"When people have a stake in something, there's no right and wrong, they just act, and that's the way it goes.

"But the times that you spent with him, I'm sure our pretty fine memories.

Yes, the experiences with Ben encompassed essentially the only book I hadn't written, and that was only he said he was going to write that book...

Sam offered his interpretation of the nightmares he'd been having.

"It just seems that the people around me have issues or needs or problems, I should say," he began, "and I've been feeling the pressure of their pressures, and I'm going to see if I can't get away from that. Because that's an infinite thing, and if ever there's an infinite issue, as long as there are people, they will always have issues, and you can't carry their issues on your shoulders. And that's what my dreams are all about: trying to help people, and it's just impossible to do.

"And so, I just have to move on with myself. And that's what I'm trying to do right now, it's not being involved in people and issues as much, and I'm just trying to wean myself off from that."

He said he was doing his exercises and trying to work on his lethargy.

"And doing my exercises, I realize that my body has really deteriorated to a point that even doing a slight exercise is a huge, huge, difficult task. So, I just have to do it very easily. Make these simple movements and build the muscle slowly, and hope that if I do it enough times, it will begin to add up, and I'll get stronger, and get more endurance.

"So, that's my plan," he concluded…

In the background, Cat Chow was becoming impatient for me to give her a treat, meowing so loud that Sam could hear her over the phone.

"It sounded like a little baby," Sam commented.

More than a baby, I rather regarded cat Chow as having become the reincarnation of my mother.

"You have your chance of giving her milk and cookies," Sara interjected in the background.

I explained to Sam how it was that all through my upbringing, my mother told me that she always wanted a mother who would wait for her at the door with milk and cookies, as opposed to the mother who she had, who was always out smoking and playing cards with the girls.

Cat Chow had even developed a hoarse voice like my mother and listening, it was as though she were saying, "Michael, how about my milk and cookies now?"

"'Well, it's about time'," Sam added, humorously.

Yes, it was about time that I'd acted like the good Japanese son that my mother wanted me to be. Someone like Sam.

"You give me too much credit," Sam said. "It's cool that you think in that manner. It makes the chore of doing things a little bit more acceptable and exciting."

Yes, a lot more fun.

"The more reason that you can give yourself to do something, the better," he declared. "It's really interesting that we've come up with such an analogies and metaphors in what we do and how we do it. I think it's actually a very important aspect of why we do things…"

Sam asked about our plans for the rest of the day? I said that we were about to walk out the door to get a falafel and asked if we could get him involved? Bring him a falafel? Take him out for a falafel?

But he declined, insisting that he wanted to get to his exercises.

"I find when I feel the motivation to do something, I got to do it," he said. "Because I find it so easy to just sit down and close my eyes and lay still and feel like I'm normally breathing. Versus trying to do something and strain for every breath. So, since I feel like straining myself a little bit, I should take advantage of that."

I told him to let me know if he thought I could be helpful.

"I was thinking about that today," he said. "I was thinking that, overall, your external Qi Gong has been very helpful for me. I remember those times with my headaches and my hand shaking when I got rid of those things. And even overall, I think you always gave me a little boost of energy after your sessions and that sort of made me relax and regain and reenergized me. It's sort of like plugging in a charger and feeling the battery charge go up a little bit. So, it's always been at the minimum that way. At its best, it turned things around. Like the headache, my shaking, a lethargy I was feeling, and various pains in the body. With those things, it has been very, very useful and helpful. That's why I always think that, 'Yeah, there's a place for this in medicine, and if you can hone it in even better, you might be able to show tremendous results, even beyond the results that you've gone so far.'

"It will just take some work. There's something there, and it just needs to be put into a more disciplined manner. So that you can say, 'Yeah, do this and you get that', rather than saying, 'Well, we do this and you get what you need.' I keep thinking there's a little bit more than just getting what you need. But maybe pushing it to a thing where you get what you need plus something more - And I think that 'plus more', you're right at the verge of doing."

"The other thought I had before we end this conversation is, you're working on me, and I'm declining. So, there is an end point with me that's within a foreseeable future. Just like with Ethel. That was the first book I read. Because she was also at a late stage, even worse than me. And so, bioenergy is of value, but that's not what your main course is. Your main course is helping people while they're still viable and are just having a little bit more than a hiccup in their lives - but it's a severe hiccup they can't overcome easily, and you make it possible for them to overcome that, and that to me is the most important aspect of what you can offer.

"I mean, it's nice that you can do things for people like me, but really, I'm not the key subject who is the most important. It's people like Ruth, your brother, Whitney, and other people who just need to overcome various things that I would say are more 'temporary.'

"People might not think it's temporary, but in reality, when you look at it, they will get through it with your help, and then just keep

moving on with our lives and forget you. And forget the issue that they had. And they just move on with their lives."

"I think that's where your value should lie," he concluded. "In helping people get through their difficult time at the moment…"

I asked Sam if I could take him to the Rink to go skating for his birthday? He indicated that he had plans to have dinner with his wife and didn't want to put any kind of schedule.

I had to laugh, remembering a Valentines Day that I took him away from May to go skiing.

He added that he appreciated the sentiment, and we'd plan to go skating another time.

Yes, when I'd called the skating rink the day before, even the staff was anxious to wish him well...

CHAPTER SEVENTEEN

Monday, July 14, 2025

On a call with our "spirit buddy", Steve, I told him about wanting to take Sam skating, and his wanting to wait. In response, Steve described a last wish expressed by a former client.

"He had pancreatic cancer, and they were treating it with chemotherapy," he began. "But they said it was incurable, as pancreatic cancer usually is. And he wanted to go to the Outer Banks. At this point, it was April, and he wanted to spend July there with his whole family. And he was so focused on that.

"So, both he and his wife came in and said, 'What should we do?' And I said, 'You want so much to have that time, and this chemo will give you that time, so that you can have it with your family.'

"And of course, I'd left it up to him… But they were interested in my opinion, and my opinion was to complete the things with this great vacation that you're so looking forward to with your extended family.

"But, of course, what happened was, the chemo made him so sick that he had to be hospitalized after each treatment. And after about the third treatment, he was so, so ill that he said, 'I'm not doing this anymore.' And it was so sad, because he didn't get his family vacation in the Outer Banks.

"So, I was wrong, and it was a mistake. He went through a lot of torture. And I guess I didn't realize what some of the effects of the chemo can be for someone who is compromised."

Yes, I thought. But can't the medical profession tell you what you're in for? How torturous it can be?...

Still talking with Steve about Sam, I thought about those "easy-breezy" Pulmonologists who essentially shrugged off Sam and his condition.

"Well, we don't know what's going to happen," they essentially told him. "We just have to wait for the next time you have an exacerbation."

"Oh, give me a f'ing break," I thought. "He has no pulmonary reserves. The moment he has an exacerbation, he's dead and you know it! He's a set up for pneumonia, and when that happens, it's going to be really awful, and he's going to really suffer and probably die."

"Yes, I really get that," Steve said. "Because his doctors weren't telling my client anything. They were just telling him, 'It's up to you. It's your decision.'"

Just like those Stanford Pulmonologists. They offered no connection. No warmth. No depth. No connection. No care. It was just, "Let's get this over with, so we can get back to our great lives."

"I'm older and wiser now," Steve continued, "and the older and wiser me would have said to my client, 'Maybe try one treatment, and if it's horrible, and you are really, really sick afterwards, don't continue it. Your remaining life and quality of life is more important, than spending days in the hospital in excruciating pain.'"

"But at the time, I didn't know," he concluded. "I really didn't know."

I didn't think the same could be said for those Pulmonologists…

Steve harkened back to Sam's experience with lung transplant screening before being told that the results of his previous CT precluded him from that procedure all the time.

"Did they know that they weren't going to do the transplant before they started the test?" Steve, asked, in disbelief. "That is unbelievable. My God, there is no excuse."

Steve described a recent experience in which a doctor refused to answer his questions.

"It was the doctor who did my prostate biopsy," he explained. "He said, 'We can wait six months and see what your PSA is, or we can just do a biopsy.' And I said, 'Well, if this were a family member or a friend, what would you tell them based on what the PSA is right now?' And he got all upset and shouted, 'I cannot tell you. I cannot answer that. I do not answer personal questions'

"So, it's like what you need an expert for the hard questions," Steve added. "Because some doctors won't answer those questions…"

Steve inquired about Sam.

"Is he holding his own?" he asked. "I mean, is he able to breath OK? Or is it getting worse and worse?"

I said I was concerned he was getting worse, and how Sam had asked not to be the focus of my Qi Gong work and just wanted to be another person in the group.

"Oh, good God," Steve said, in despair. "I guess that's his path. I guess he's chosen his path. If I was his therapist, I would feel heartbroken. Because it is so clear to me that what you are doing with him can have really permanent changes. And we know this, because of the fact that people with terminal conditions like cancer or whatever can be changed."

"So, he's wrong," Steve concluded. "But that's what he's choosing…"

I was trying not to be judgmental and accept Sam's "path." Because, really, he was just being realistic, as staving off or reversing the disease process would mean a miracle.

But it seemed to me I'd seen miracles happen: Kino overcoming those neurologic deficits... Well, the experts said they were permanent. And like Sam, he had the CT replete with the tissue damage to show it. And yet, it happened. He did overcome those neurologic deficits with Qi Gong. It was a miracle, but it happened. So, why shouldn't Sam go for a miracle? What does he have to lose?

"Exactly," Steve said. "Exactly. Oh God, I'm totally with you. I am completely with you. 'What does he have to lose?'

"But he's sort of closing up. Closing up shop is what it sounds like. And that's very, very sad. Very sad. Because it doesn't have to be..."

He broke off.

"It's awful," he concluded.

Listening to myself, though, I knew I was wrong: For years, I'd hated when a lack of positive thinking was turned around so that when a patient didn't display it, it was used as a source of blame against the patient. And that's what I was doing! I was handling this all wrong!

Sara was right: I was blaming Sam. I had let my emotions get in the way of rational thinking. I had to pull myself back…

Steve had to get off the phone, and Sara asked me if I would join her at the Greek restaurant near Sam's?

Initially, I told her no, because I felt like Sam was telling me to stay away, and the thought of being nearby and not visiting him was too hurtful.

But ultimately, I did choose to join Sara; and then I reached out to Sam and asked if I could bring him some baklava? And he told me that was OK…

At the door, I handed Sam the baklava, and he led me inside.

"Ah, life is like being a salmon," Sam said, waxing philosophical. "You swim and swim and swim upstream to get to the spawning grounds, and then when you get there, it's like, 'Hey, I'm molting. I'm about to die.'"

He laughed.

I responded by telling him about when I was in college, I knew a couple of pre-Vet students who were so worried about a giant Koi in a campus pond that they caught the fish and injected it with penicillin to help it get better.

"I could see you doing that, Mike," he replied. "I could have seen you becoming a Veterinarian, because you care so much about animals."

I shook my head and told him that my Dean in college actually tried to sway me towards to become a veterinarian.

"You got the grades to be able to get into Vet school," the Dean said. "Have you ever considered that?"

"And spend all my time taking care of animals?" I'd responded. "That's not important. Why would I want to do that?"

"It was probably good that you didn't become a veterinarian," he said, compassionately, "because they have among the highest suicide rates of any profession. Even more than doctors, veterinarians got into their profession because they really, really care about animals. Probably more so than doctors who treat humans. Because when people have pets, they love their animals, but a lot of them don't have the money to pay for proper treatment. Or they feel that 'It's an animal. You shouldn't have to pay as much for the care of an animal as you would a human being.' So, the vet is in a quandary of saying, 'I need to take care of this animal', and they really are passionate about wanting to take care of that animal and do the right thing for the animal. But most of the patients, or the owners, don't want to pay. And, so, the vet goes in and helps their animal and usually gets short changed. Because they have to run a business, too. I mean, medicine for an animal costs pretty much the same as a human. The machinery. The instruments. The lab fees. Tests. So, they're really in

a quandary, and the anxieties and pressures, psychologically-wise, are very much higher for vets.

"And the insurance is hardly existent for pets. And when you do find insurance, the insurance companies really don't want to pay hardly at all for the treatments. So, for a vet to really maintain their practice at a real high level, a lot of them are really struggling.

"And then, a lot of times, I'm sure that the vets know that they can help and save an animal; but, a lot of times, the owners, due to cost or whatever, don't put a higher priority towards their animal pet. Of course, there are people like the Yanuck's who will do just about anything for their pet; but they're not the typical owner or significant percentage of customers for the vet. So, it's difficult for vets, unless the vet is set up a practice in a very affluent neighborhood."

"Anyway," he concluded, "that's some of the reasons that there is pressure on vets. I'm sure there are others that I haven't thought of or considered..."

Performing external Qi Gong treatment on Sam, I felt a lot of energy coming from his chest. As I followed it with my right hand, both hands became activated, and my crown chakra "popped", so to send me backwards.

Afterwards, I found myself in my own 'little bubble', while Sam was sitting some three or four feet away.

"I feel good," Sam declared. "I feel a little bit better than before we started. My chest is a little bit lighter. Not as heavy."

"The interesting thing is, Mike," he continued, "when you do these sessions, there's the immediate feeling that I get - A feeling of being lighter and less burdened - And what is good is it kind of goes for a while like that. So, it has a bit of a residual effect, so that it makes me feel good for a while."

Earlier, Sam had talked about having significant difficulties in the mornings, so I hoped the effect of the treatment would linger till then.

"Don't press your luck," Sam responded, doubtful.

He laughed.

"It's something that we wish for, of course," he added. "We'll see. We'll see when I wake up.

"But if I can get to sleep... Well, that's important. Period. But I tell you, I'm getting some weird dreams. Nightmares, actually. For instance, I'm having these dreams of going to college, and it's my last year, and I have to complete these courses, and it's finals this week, so I'm going to have to take a final in these classes, and I go, 'I haven't been attending this class. I don't know what's going to be in

the final.' And then I get panicky, and I think, 'Shit, what have I been doing all this time?'

"And then, for another dream, I'll be in a different class, and I study the wrong thing, and I'm super panicking, going, 'I'm not going to graduate. I'm failing. And I don't know what to do.' And I'm thinking about my family, and it's worse than death, because there's this thing about failing: Failing to me is so worse than death. It's like you don't have a soul if you fail. It's like you're nobody. And it's in your dream, so all of these emotions are being amplified. You're adrenaline is up. And it's really, really bad. That's one pack of dreams.

"The other dreams are not so much about me. In fact, in the dream, I'm really healthy. I'm perfect health wise. Normal. But all around me are people who have problems, anxieties, health issues, personal issues, depression, psychosis, everything. And it's like being in a black-and-white movie, and all I see are shades of gray… No color. No color at all. And I'm in a tidal pool, and it's just kind of hazy and all gray and cloudy, and you just see people walking through the tide pools, and they're just these depressed, anxiety-ridden people, like zombies - Just walking. That's all I see. And these people are just everywhere. It's just a sea of these people that goes on forever and ever and ever. And the further you look, the more people you see who are distressed. And I'm just going, 'This is like a living hell.' And they're just sucking the life force out of you. Because you can't do anything for them - They're just past the point of no return. And they're right there upon your knees. They're all over the place. And it's so dreary and damp and just so terrible. And I'm in the middle of it. Anyway, that's another type of dream.

"And then there's another type of dream series: I'm with a bunch of people who are committing crimes. And I don't know: Apparently I'm part of it. They're a gang. Or they're a group. and I'm in their car, and we're running around, and either being chased or going to do some hijacking or criminal act. And I'm trying to convince them not to do it, or if we have to do something that's a criminal act, we shouldn't hurt anyone while we're doing it - to keep them from doing something really harmful. And I'm just kind of trapped in that scenario, and I don't know what's going to happen? Is someone going to get killed? Or maybe I'll get killed? And we're just going on and on. And at certain points I'm thinking, 'Well, I'm going to change them.' Then, another time, I'm thinking, 'Oh, it's hopeless, they're turning against me.' And it's just this point when you're right on the edge that you don't know what's going to happen - Your life is at risk, or someone else's life is at risk? It's just that pressure there…"

Sam offered his interpretation of the last series of dreams.

"My body is this vehicle that I'm trapped in," he explained, "with bad things in my body that are going to do whatever they want. So, I have no control. I have no control of myself. I've lost all my control physically right now. And I'll be losing it mentally soon. My dreams know exactly what I'm going through."

"The problem is," he continued, "with some of these dreams, you wake up, but you think you're still in it. And before it used to be that I would wake up from a nightmare, and I'd go, 'Oh, it's only a dream' and you move on. But nowadays, I wake up, and I'm going, 'I'm still in it. I'm awake, but I'm still in it.' And I'm going, 'Oh, shit. I gotta get ready for the test.' Then I go, 'What test? Where is it going to be? I can't find the room.' And I'm awake, yet I'm having these thoughts, so it's not like I feel that these are dreams. I feel like I'm still in them. And I'm still participating. And it takes me a while to just calm down and regroup, till I start going, 'Did I graduate? I think I have a diploma somewhere in the house.' Then, I realize, 'Well, yeah, I have a diploma. I, I, I passed.' But up to that point, I was freaking out - even though I wasn't dreaming. Man, that takes a lot out of you. And you think you're going crazy.

"So, this is what happens when you're in a state that you're not healthy. To the point that it's irreversible. you're only going to go one direction.

"And even when you talk to people who are going through similar things. Like I was in a group chat with other people having lung issues, and they talk about their situation, which are similar to mine. None of them are going to get lung transplants. and they're having similar difficulties as I am. And so, what they're trying to do is see if they can live with it every day with their condition and try to optimize their life, just like what I'm doing.

"But in my opinion, there's really only one way to escape this. And so, yes, I might be able to make it through another day, but I'm not going to escape this. Because I'll eventually die.

"So, that's one thing you should not do - Is think of it that way. Because then your mind keeps focusing on that one door, and then you don't optimize your life that you're currently living. And when you know that today is the best day of your future, if you don't optimize it, you lose it. Because you're not going to ever have that opportunity today, because the next day you're going to have some other issues, which you have to try to optimize on top of the other ones that are failing.

"So, you shouldn't be thinking about... Well, you understand what I'm saying... You cannot be wasting your time thinking about the other things, except for how to optimize your current thing. But you're losing so many points that you don't have any points left to play with? It's sort of like a poker game... You start to say, 'I really have no more money to throw into the pot, because I keep drawing up short. I'm still playing, because I still have some coins, and I'm playing and thinking, 'Maybe I'll get lucky', and, 'Maybe you might win a minor game, so that you got some more points, to extend things a little bit longer'..."

I told Sam that I thought he was putting a lot of pressure on himself.

"Yeah, I know," he said. "And if I'm not doing it consciously, it's coming out subconsciously in my dreams. And that's really tough, too - trying to change. How do you change your dream patterns? I think there is a way, but I haven't figured it out.

"And I think, 'If I think of really, really happy thoughts... Well, where is Mary Poppins when you need her? There's no spoonful of sugar..."

Sam commented about history.

"If you look at history, there are periods where civilization is really good. And then you have periods that are really bad, like Nazi Germany... Can you think of anything worse?

"And then, you have other periods and other empires, where, oh my goodness, you look at India and the temples that are found in the jungles, and the walls are very low - There were no walls fortification.

"But of course, that civilization is gone and in ruins, but before it went into that dismal state, it flourished with grandeur."

"So, like I said," he concluded, "it all depends on when you were born..."

I commented that I felt the baby boomers had it pretty good when it came to opportunity.

As for me, I felt my life changed with proposition 13, when the government stopped being as generous to students.

Still, I felt I had it a lot better than today's kids, when it came to reasonable tuition, reasonable rent, reasonable travel fares. I could work my minimum wage job and pay for college.

"That's because there was a lot of infrastructure that supported that," Sam responded. "Small businesses could thrive.

"Today, there are cameras everywhere, so that people have to act a certain way. We're being controlled. People are being manipulated. Online dating. They match you. It's really, really weird, Michael. There's so much marketing. The freedom is shrinking. We're talking about a grim future. There was a huge population that voted for Obama that now votes for Trump. How do you figure that? How can you get people who voted for Obama to switch over and vote for Trump? Because of social media manipulation of the Internet search. Weaponizing certain groups: Megachurches using the words of Jesus Christ and the word of God for their own purposes - to gather sheep for their flock, so that they could gain power. The church makes Jesus seem like a person who wants power. How does somebody who sacrificed as much as he did be made to want power? It doesn't make sense."

"The point is, Mike," he concluded, "the world is screwed up and it's getting worse, but the control is really interesting..."

I told Sam that my prescription to him was, in this screwed up world where people have decided to choose fear over courage, to go out and be with people, just like the way he was at the Stanford emergency department, and made everyone feel so appreciated, and change the world just through his genuine goodness and positivity.

"I hope I can do it," he said. "It feels overwhelming."

I thought that was the source of his dreams. Feeling like a failure because the bleakness in the world just made it all so impossible to help others, especially at this time when his strength was at a minimum...

Sam said that he was practicing roller-skating, so that he could go to the Rink one more time.

I said that if you wanted to practice at the rink, I would be happy to take him, even if he was only able to go a quarter of a lap.

"I was really appreciative that you would do that for me on my birthday," he said. "Except that I'm not ready yet."

Whenever you're ready, I told him.

"Yes, I'm getting there, because it gives me a goal to improve my health, because I want to go skating," he said. "And maybe I can go skating, at least one more time, so that I could have a good time."

I thought he would have a good time no matter what. Just being there and seeing people, I thought he would have a good time.

"Yeah, I know I would," he responded. "I think there's still time for me.

"And we gotta do it before you go to back East. Hopefully, sooner than later."

Sam reminisced about when I was just a guy that he enjoyed talking with at the rollerskating rink

"And then you talked about bioenergy, and I was really intrigued," he said…

As I was about to leave, he said that he was looking forward to eating the baklava that I brought as a belated birthday gift.

Then, he told me that he appreciated me coming over and hoped that he didn't waste too much of my time, and I lost it.

"Are you kidding, Sam?" I said, my whole body slumping and chest caving in upon itself. "God Almighty, I live to be with you."

"I appreciate that," he responded. "But you're a busy guy, and I don't want to be taking up too much of your time. Thank you very much..."

CHAPTER EIGHTEEN

Tuesday, July 15, 2025.

Driving near Sam's, I asked if he'd like some more baklava? He declined the baklava, but said he would like me to visit.

At his home, I performed Qi Gong. Scanning him, I experienced a number of energy vortices coming from his chest and directed at my right hand. The vortices were moving in a counterclockwise direction as they made contact with my hand, and it was like nothing I've ever experienced before. The energy from the vortices directed me upwards towards Sam's crown chakra, and as I followed it, my crown chakra popped.

Then, the energy guided me around Sam, circling him over and over, moving from a higher level of his body, to a lower level; and the end was so definite, like one moment I was feeling the vortex, and the next, it was all gone, and there was nothing but air there.

But a moment later, to my surprise, I was feeling the vortex out my hand, but instead of coming from Sam, there was some reversal, and they were coming out from me, and in this case, they were moving in the clockwise direction.

And the place in my hand where I was feeling this reverse vortex was that same as where it had been hit by Sam's energy; that being, in the space between my thumb and index finger along the lateral aspect of my palmar surface.

Then, the energy took me back to Sam to perform Qi emission; and I noticed that my chest was wide open, and there was nothing sunken and concave about it. None of the usual tightness - Like it was just relaxed.

Sam had been quiet for a long time, then finally spoke.

"Thanks, Mike," he said. "What I felt for me, after you were done and told me, 'Feel free to do what you want', I felt like your energy was still working on me, and that there was a pressure inside my chest cavity pushing outwards and trying to expand my chest - which is good, because it's like trying to make room against this different strain that feels restricting and is usually painful. But this one is pushing out and feeling like a balloon trying to make space for my lungs."

"So, it feels like there's tension, but it's good tension," he concluded. "And that feeling of tightness is more like stretching - the way I need it. I haven't felt that before."

He got up from the chair and said he felt like performing the evening Qi Gong exercise with Lee Holden.

"I feel like I have the energy for it," he said.

I asked if I could join him, and we performed it together…

Leaving Sam's house, I decided to take a walk around Curtis Park, near his home.

Then, a minute or so into my walk, Sam called to tell me more about the way he was feeling after the external Qi Gong treatment.

"When you were doing it, my chest seemed to be pushing outwards from inside," he said. "Well, I think that kind of helped me when we did the internal Qi Gong with Lee Holden, because I didn't feel any stress in my chest while we were doing it. I felt tired in other ways, but not with the compression feeling at the chest, which was kind of interesting, and I just realized that. So, I think there was a correlation. I just wanted to let you know that…"

Arriving home, Sara commented about Sam's dreams and the experiences that he was having with them, feeling like he was still in them.

"So, he is entering the spirit dream and recognizing that it's a different state of being, and therefore it kind of registers as a dream state," she said. "I don't know if it's true or not?"

I didn't think that the spirit world would be so scary?

"Oh, because he's having all of those fears," she responded. "I guess we should all hope that that's not what the spirit world is like."

Yes, that certainly was not what I would be anticipating.

Then again, though, maybe that's why spirits are willing to take the plunge into the physical world? They have some motivation, because the spirit world isn't exactly heaven...

CHAPTER NINETEEN

Wednesday, July 16, 2025

While performing external Qi Gong with Sam, he offered his interpretation of the dream with the guys in the car.

"My body is this vehicle that I'm trapped in, with bad things in my body they are going to do whatever they want to do," he began. "So, I have no control. I have no control of myself. I've lost all my control physically right now. And I'll be losing it mentally soon. My dreams know exactly what I'm going through."

Energetically, I'd been receiving energy with my right hand from his chest at the time, that took my hand towards my right chest, so that the two were interacting energetically. Energy came into my left hand, and my crown chakra got activated. Meanwhile, the energy in my right hand, followed a path back to Sam, so to perform Qi emission back at Sam's chest. And then the energy took me around and around Sam in a clockwise direction, with energy being emitted from my right hand.

Meanwhile, my left hand was interacting with my solar plexus chakra, which was activated. Then, the energy left my hands, though my solar plexus and Crown chakra remained activated.

Sam described feeling like there was no certainty that he would wake up in the morning.

"I'm trying to get to a state where I don't worry about that," he said. "I never did that before. I never worried about stepping out of the house in a car running me over. So, why should I worry about these things until they happen? I say that to myself, but saying something to yourself and doing it are two separate things."

He talked about the belief in God.

"It's so nice to believe that there's somebody who can help you," he began. "Like when I was a little kid, even though my dad was stern and very disciplined, whenever I needed help, he was the kindest, tenderness person. He was always there for me. Just like my mom. She was always kind. She was not stern. Even when she was stern, you knew that she wasn't."

"My dad, though, when he was stern, he was stern!" he clarified. "Anyway, I always had someone who I could think and ask for help when I was a kid. So, when you don't have a parent, that's when God comes in.

"Like, when something good happens, I go, 'Thank God.' But there's probably no God up there that listens or heard that. But I have to thank somebody. I can't say, 'Thank Mike Yanuck.' But God has some more meaningful attachment in relation to that.

"And then, when you need help, you pray to God. Even though, most of the time, it's not going to help you. Look at all the people who prayed for God to help them in disastrous times, and you go to the survivors, and they'll tell you that God helped them - Because they asked if God's help. But those are the survivors. Try asking a dead person, 'Did God help you?'"

Yes, I'd always thought of the 6 million of my brethren who were murdered in the concentration camps and imagined every last one of them was praying to God at the moment that they were gassed to death.

"But people will tell you that God has his reasons," Sam continued. "So, I catch myself when I say, 'Thank God.' But it makes me feel good, so I still will continue, though it doesn't mean I want to. It's more of a reaction for me than expecting something."

He talked about the help that he received from his mother and father when he was sick.

"They would get water for me, or an ice pack," he said. "That was tangible. But when there's no one around you who can give you that, then you go for God, because it's in your mind and it will give you some relief."

"I think there is something, but it's in your mind," he asserted. "And some people will go, 'No, it's not in your mind - It's actually God putting that in your mind."

"Anyway, we'll see if I end up at the pearly gates. Or maybe not. But either place, it's going to be heavily populated with souls. So, I'll be asking, 'Is there any room for me here? It just seems like there's a hell of a lot of souls here: People souls and animal souls, and you're just going, 'Get this monkey off my back.'"

"But it's all a human construct," he concluded…

I confided that I wondered that this energy we were working with wasn't connected to some "higher power"? I'd been taught that it was connected with the "Universal Qi", which served as a universal blueprint to tap into and facilitate the healing of all things for the return of function to extent possible for a person. And when I worked with this energy, it led me to feel there was some energetic connection happening that was consistent with what I'd been taught.

"But is it just for physical people?" Sam asked. "Or is it also for people after death? Does it go beyond that? Just because you can't see it, you can't smell it, you can't hear it, you can't taste it, doesn't mean it's not there. Or does it somehow embrace everyone's soul to make it more powerful? So that maybe the Qi is a vampire that sucks its energy from living beings? You never know where energy is? If you believe in the conservation of energy, that you cannot create energy, nor can you destroy it, then energy just is, and it gets transferred into another form of energy, and at this point in time, it's very important for living people."

I commented about love energy being one that is not only recyclable, but also, self-propagating. The only source of energy I know like that is love. When you love someone, it grows and snowballs and spreads one to another, such that I believe that's where our hope as a species lies.

"I find that love is an energy that just works in a more kinder, gentler way," Sam responded. "Like it takes energy. And I think love takes energy from hate. Because when you love something, it's hard to hate it. So, that energy of hate gets transformed into love. So, it's a damn good form of energy. Because I think a lot of people put a lot of energy into hate. And when they hate, there's not as much love there.

"I think that's the wonderful thing about a human being… That a human being can direct these things.

"Now there are flawed human beings like psychopaths, who can't have empathy or love or kindness. So, what's that?"

I thought that was a problem of wiring in the brain, though it did lead me to wonder what occurred for a state of being in which there wasn't a brain (like the spirit state)?

"Anyway, a lot of questions to answer," he concluded…

"These questions are not new for me," Sam continued. "I've been thinking about these things ever since I was a child. I went to Christian churches when I was really young and saw people who worship Jesus Christ, who had a strong faith.

"And I went to the Buddhist church, as well, and met good people there, too. And then I had my Jewish friends and their commitment and going to the synagogues and all that. But I think I've been jaded, because everyone I've met have been really great people. Kind people. Wise people.

"But there were always a few outliers, and that's what intrigued me - the outliers. Why did they behave in a certain way and why were they so destructive?"

Because they were human, I responded.

As for me, my questions about this life and hereafter had been answered thirty years ago in the defining event that determined my spirituality:

It happened at my friend Wah's house: He, Elizabeth and I would get together on the weekends to practice Qi Gong in his basement; but on this occasion, I was tired, so when the two of them got up to practice, I told them to go on without me.

Then, just as they were about to start, Elizabeth turned and said, 'Mike, watch my aura.'

I'd had a couple experiences seeing auras, and said I would, then sat back on the couch.

They began to practice, and – sure enough – I saw Liz's aura. It looked like this thick film of buzzy gray stuff coming off all around her.

In turn, she was patting herself, starting at her head, to her shoulders, then torso, and this gray film seems to be moving down into the ground.

'Good,' I thought, watching. 'She's probably getting rid of a lot of bad energy – turbid Qi. I bet she's going to feel a lot better after this.'

Then - out of nowhere - there's this burst of white light that flashed from her! Just for a second - Bang! - like a firefly or quick explosion!

I was thrown back against the couch by the pure emotional impact of what I'd seen.

Whoa?! I thought. What was that?!'

Elizabeth was even more affected and visibly trembling all over. Looking afraid and seemingly unable to speak, she beckoned me with her hands to come to her. Arriving at her side, she told me to hold her - Wah, too – saying she felt cold and seen something that scared her.

Then, she told us her vision: She saw herself carrying a dead body from a past life to a lot of otherworldly creatures that took the body, then told her to go back to her life.

Hence, this was the defining event that determined my spirituality. From this experience (between what I saw and what Elizabeth described) I hold that, at its core, life is about a spirit entity learning the lessons of the universe on the physical plane.

"You don't need a spacecraft," Sam responded...

It was time for the meeting of the Qi Gong group, and Sam and I sat, and I started the computer. I began by apologizing for last week when I'd let my brother speak so long and offered my reasons and concluded by saying that that wouldn't happen again.

I announced that Sam did not want to be the focus of the self-practice and want everybody to be involved and share their experiences.

I shared that Sam had a really hard day with pulmonary rehab, so we wouldn't be staying on too long.

With that, we began to the self-practice. Interestingly, the Qi in the ball of energy exercise brought my hands very close to each other, though they never touched each other.

Finally, my hands spread apart, so that they were palms up, and my crown chakra very activated.

I shared how it was that I was learning that the hands are associated with the heart chakra and Heart Meridian and left me feeling like this exercise offered a balance of the head and the heart.

My hands were brought downward in a convoluted movement that was different from the usual simple bending at the elbows and then remained rather levitated above my lap, and it seemed that the energy was going to keep them there.

I found that my higher third eye was very activated. I took time to just sit in the energy, with hands, radiating energy and energy in my crown chakra.

Finally, after the energy had left my hands, so I felt very strongly in my higher third eye. I suppose it made sense with all the talking that Sam and I had been doing about spirituality versus living in the world. The third eye is where you integrate that experience, interfacing between the divine energy with all of its altruism and love, and the chakras below that we're all about survival. Hence, we were integrating our altruistic, divine nature, with those elements that we need to live in the world, and the two could become conflicted when you're between your altruistic nature and your survival one.

Interestingly, as I spoke, most of the energy moved to my crown chakra.

I turned to Sam and asked how he was doing?

"Yes, I'm doing fine," he responded. "It was actually quite interesting for me. It started off with energy in the hands. Then, it moved throughout my arms and legs, my upper body into my head. Today it didn't seem like the hands were the centerpiece, but my whole body. I feel this buzzing throughout my whole body. And it kind of made me feel better, because slightly I've been having all kinds of weakness throughout the body. So maybe the energy started in the hands, but then wanted to distribute energy throughout the whole body to get the body some life energy, so that I could continue to move about.

"So, that's my take: It wasn't just in the hands, but it moved throughout the whole body. In the legs, even in my feet and toes. So, I felt this lively buzzing throughout the body. So, it was a good experience…"

After Sam shared his experience, he actively engaged the others, offering responses for their Qi experiences.

"I had a little bit of a different experience," Ruth offered. "Initially, I was holding my hands, 8 inches apart, feeling the breeze between the two hands, but eventually I felt a need to touch my face and different areas where I had medical procedures, so that it was more of a touching experience then just an energy from a little bit away. So, I'm not sure if it was Qi Gong or not? It was different."

"I think it's really important that the greater the understanding of that," Sam responded, "and Mike has experienced quite a bit with his modality and that makes him quite powerful in that area."

Ruth added that after she was done with her practice, she had an interesting interaction with her cats.

"My kitties came over one at a time and wanted me to pet them from head to tail," she said. "And then they both left. So my question is, Does this work on kitties too?"

"Yes, animals have a feeling for sensing cheese that we don't have," Sam asserted and commented about the migration of birds. "They arrive at a certain place at the right time, so they're capable of understanding electromagnetic forces, and I imagine other animals have that, as well..."

CHAPTER TWENTY

Sunday, July 20, 2025

Sam complained that his doctors were less than caring, comparing the way he works with clients in his ski school to the way he was treated by them.

"These are people who have so many other things that they can put their energy into," he said. "But right now they're just so focused: 'I really wanna improve my skiing. I really want to have some fun.' So, for me, if it's possible, I'm going to put everything I can into giving them that hope that they can improve and show them that they can do it. And it won't be that difficult. It's within their reach. And that's all I can think about for this person.

"And after their first session with me, they're usually like, 'Oh my God. I learned so much in this 30, 40 minutes than I have all the years that I've been skiing.' And then they feel hope and they ask, 'How often should I come back?'

"And I don't even need to know their name. Your name is just a label anyways. So, I don't remember my students' names. But I do remember their enthusiasm, their passion, and what they need to get to the next stage.

"But I don't feel that from my doctors and people, in general. It feels like this world is full of dead fishes. It's like shaking their hand, and their hand is so limp that they're just sticking it out there. It used to not be that way. It used to be that when someone said something, they really meant it. These days, people go, 'Yeah', and tell me how important their work is; but they never get around to it. Versus people in the past who delivered.

"For example, if someone ever needed some money, I lent it, because I knew that they would pay it back. Now, you give it to them, you don't expect to ever see it.

"Even my rollerskates: I just gave them away to Escape Club. And the person said, 'Oh, this is fabulous. I'm going to give you a donation card number, so that you can write them off on your taxes'; but he never sent it to me. Again, people's words, even for something as simple as that… Well, they know it's no sweat off their back to keep their promises. There's no integrity…"

I shared that the other day I'd been out with Dino; he'd confided that his girlfriend had suggested that he was somehow autistic; I, on the other hand, wondered that I was neurotic?

"Why do you think that you're neurotic?" Sam asked. "What did you do that was neurotic? Or would be labeled neurotic? Were you collecting certain things?"

I said that when I would visit a friend's family (I didn't say Bubbles, because Sam had previously indicated he preferred to avoid other's personal issues), I would stay at their house. And when one of their daughters got married, I still expected that, to the point that when they didn't make those accommodations available to me, I asked if I should bring a tent and sleep in the backyard? And it didn't ever enter my mind to stay at a hotel, and wouldn't that be considered weird?

"I don't think that was weird," Sam said. "Comparing the family you wanted to stay with to your family, did you enjoy their family interaction more than the interactions you had with your own family?"

So much more: Bubbles's mother was warm and loving; her father engaged me in conversation, whereas mine would only humiliate me.

"OK, I would've guessed that," Sam said. "And that's all you wanted: In your mind, you're saying, 'I like this family interaction. I want to be part of that. I want to feel like family. To me, in my mind, this is what a family should be. Because this is my ideal family', or, 'This is not ideal, but it's way, way significantly better than the family environment that I have.'

"So, yeah, I see that. You wanted to be close. It's sort of like a child craving for a specific toy: They love firetrucks; but their parent never gave them a firetruck. And the child goes to a friend's house, and he sees a firetruck, and you want it. And sometimes, you might want to take it home with you; and for some reason, it just overrides the feeling of what you believe is being polite, because it's one thing to say, 'Can I borrow it for right now and play with it, and then I'll give it back to you?' But you're so deprived that you hold onto it, and it becomes yours, because you feel safe with it and secure.

"So, of course you want to take it. And you start walking out the door with it when it's time to leave, and then they say, 'Oh, you've got to give this back.' It happens to so many kids.

"So, you were just wanting something. And although this doesn't offer an explanation for all of it, it explains the desire.

"And that isn't neuroticism. That's normality. You know how many kids do that and how many people wish for something that they're lacking? It's like, if you're missing a vitamin for normal function, then you start searching out food that makes you feel better, because it contains that nutrient that you're lacking. It's a survival mechanism: You're missing something that's really essential to normality - To a balance. So, of course you're going to crave it. The more you're missing it and deficient in it, the stronger the urge."

As he spoke, I remembered the dream I'd had on Bubbles' birthday and the letter I'd written her about it:

I dreamt about your mother: We were at the house (though it was different and looked larger and more expansive and ornate). She was talking with someone about me (though I don't know to whom), saying, "He isn't a 50-50 guy. He doesn't do anything halfway. He puts his whole heart into everything he does. And when he would visit, it wasn't like he couldn't afford a hotel; he stayed with us, because he wanted to be a part of us..."

Then, I remembered Bubbles' telling me that I was like family to her:

"When I think about you, it's like a brother - I want to know where you are..."

I was making plans for my mother's burial. In the family plot, there were three gravesites left. I wanted my mother to be buried next to my grandfather, but my mother had asked that my craven brother make the arrangements for her, and I choose to honor that, because my awful uncle wanted to be buried there side-by-side with his wife, and the only two spaces like that were next to my grandfather, my mother would be buried somewhere else in the plot. And, as a result, my mother would not be buried next to my grandfather, and my awful uncle and his wife would have the last two places, so that I could not be buried in the family plot.

But at the same time, I think maybe he was doing me a favor, and, "Is that really the place where you feel like you'd find a lot of peace? That you would 'rest in peace'? With this family that left you feeling so deprived and 'deficient' and cheated? I think you'd probably find more peace somewhere else?"

"Yeah," Sam said. "Or just die in the woods and let the animals scatter your remains everywhere and return back to the world."

Though I found the image somewhat gruesome, this was the way that our Northern Cheyenne healer friend, phillip whiteman, suggested for our dog, Ini - which we would have pursued had it not been for my mother's passing, so that we had to attend to her estate, instead of attending Ini.

"Yes, no matter how it is," Sam continued, "whether it's scavengers or whatever, eventually it's all 'dust to dust.'

"I never understood why we have to put people in coffins? I guess it's an Egyptian thing to do. That's even worse if you ask me when it comes to Egyptians: 'Yeah, let's try to preserve them for as long as we possibly can, so that 200 or 300 or 500 years from now, people unearth it, and take off the bandages.'"

I commented that when I was young and watched the movie, "Exodus", I like the way that they buried young Jewish woman, and the Arab man, just using the equivalent of a burlap sack to enclose their bodies and then put them into the ground (Though I did have the irrational issue of feeling like that wouldn't give me a lot of ability to breathe), because it would make it easier for me to dissolve into the Earth.

"I think the Indians had it right when they put their dead on a scaffold, so that eventually everything just falls apart, but, in between, people could come and see the body in the equivalent of an open casket," Sam responded. "In this way, when people have to travel a long way to pay their respect, the memorial is longer.

"It's interesting the way people treat their dead in their ceremonies. Give you an idea of their mentality: 'Oh, we have to put you in a tomb. And by the way, we're going to kill all the servants, so that they can serve you after your dead. We'll bury everybody in the tomb with you.'

"A bit more humane was when the Chinese would just make ceramic figures. And each one was different, because it represented a different person. It was really good for the economy. It keeps pottery people in business. That's a pretty big burial plot, so you have to pay a lot of money for that..."

I asked if he wanted to do some bioenergy and Qi Gong? We went to his living room, where the massage table was already out, where he would lay on his abdomen and his wife would apply a percussive device to his mid and upper back to help clear his lungs. Now, he laid on his back.

Working with Sam energetically turned out to be a very unusual experience for me, in that I experienced these 'competing energies', which I don't think I ever experienced before.

I began by feeling the energy around his right chest with my right hand that was taking me clockwise around the table around his head and to his left side, when I found that my hand was hit by this whirling energy that spiraled up from him and directed me downwards.

And then it happened again, this time around Sam's right hip? This spiraling energy. What in the world?

In retrospect, the only time I've ever encountered anything close to spiraling energy was when I worked with chakras that needed to be realigned.

And that spiraling energy had a quality to it unlike what I was used to: Whereas before, I could flow with the energy path (Indeed, these days it was just a matter of 'plugging into' someone's energy body with essentially no need to follow anything), with this energy spiral, it was insistent that I be very specific and follow it exactly. It was like going back in time, when I was training with Bruce Rind, and I'd follow the energy, millimeter by millimeter. That's what this felt like.

And encountering the spiraling energy kept happening! The next time, the spiraling energy would direct me upwards and activate my crown chakra, and activate my left hand with healing energy, as well. The energy directed my left hand upwards to interact with the left side of my head and it felt like it was emitting healing energy towards my left temple and kept my hand there.

Meanwhile, my right hand was being directed towards Sam for Qi emission to his right chest. And then to his left chest.

Of note, Sam had been coughing, his breathing labored just before the treatment; but almost immediately from the time I interacted with him energetically, his coughing stopped and his breathing considerably eased.

At near four minutes into the treatment, the energy left my left hand, so to release that interaction at my left temple, though both my left hand and my left temple area were still charged with energy.

My right hand was still being directed around Sam, and there were still the encounters with that spiraling energy coming from him.

I was moving around and around the table, and these spiraling energy vortices were just coming out of nowhere, again and again.

Finally, the energy was directing me downward towards the ground, until the energy was out of my right hand, and I was sent in a kneeling position next to Sam on his left side, with energy at my crown chakra and even more at my left temple.

Again, where Sam had made it clear that he couldn't handle the difficulties of others right now, I tried to subdue my inclination to share. But then, I remembered Sam's comment about "firetrucks" and commented about how it was that another boy in the neighborhood where I'd grown up had thrown a firetruck at my left temple, which resulted in a head injury with residual pain and ache that bothered me for years, so that I wondered if today's energy experience there was related?

"Were you beaten up a lot when you were growing up?" Sam asked.

I didn't know that it was 'a lot'? I had my scrapes, but didn't know that it was abnormal? A neighborhood kid pushed me into an ottoman while playing hide-and-go-seek that resulted in a laceration across the right side of my forehead that had to be stitched up. Another kid would squeeze the back of my neck. Did that sound so abnormal?

"To be honest with you, yes," Sam responded. "Sounds like you were bullied, and people were picking on you. I didn't have that problem. The people I hung around with were all people who tried to help me, or work with me, or have fun when we do things. They taught me a lot, and showed me a lot of wonderful things. We liked to play and it was very mutual. It never felt like I was a subordinate or a leader. we just did things together. I know whenever I pushed someone to do something they wouldn't want to do.

"There were times when I thought, 'I don't know if this is a good thing to do.' There were always those few things that you sort of experimented with the gray areas. But if we did go into an area that had problems, no one ever bailed on you. We would always take responsibility. If we did something bad, we all took the blame together. No one ever threw anyone under the bus."

Perhaps I was bullied, but I could say this: For any mistreatment that I might have received at the hands of my "friends", it never came anywhere near the kind of abuse that I suffered at the hands of family.

"Sure," Sam said. "But that doesn't mean that the bullying wasn't bad. It was just relative. Like the way stealing is better than murder."

Again, I tried to resist the urge to talk about Bubbles, because I didn't want to burden him. But I decided to share that all those "friends" evaporated away and disappeared after my relationship with Bubbles. It was just such a different experience with her that it left me completely without any need or desire to continue my friendships with those I knew in high school; after the experience with pebbles, these high school friends had no importance or value to me anymore.

"Right," Sam said. "That's the difference that someone who cares about you will definitely make you feel. And that's important…"

He broke off.

"It's kind of sad that you felt you weren't getting the care at home or the people close to you that you needed," he continued, "and it took someone who really went out of their way to care for you - Which was Bubbles. And that's a good thing. At least you were able to get it. Just think if pebbles never came into your life? What type of person would you be today?"

"Did it change the way you behaved?" he asked. "Would you have been a little bit more of a colder fish without Bubbles? Probably so, if you ask me. Because you wouldn't know what real caring was. And so, I think pebbles showed you how to care, and take that to other people, as well, in a good way. It's like making friends. Were you able to make better and stronger friends after Bubbles?"

Of course. I knew what it was to be with someone who loved me.

"Right," Sam responded. "So, wasn't it Bubbles who was a milestone or a turning point in your life?... Yeah, you wouldn't be who you are today if it wasn't for Bubbles. Maybe it would have come at a different time and in a different way, because you always had it in you. It's just that she just brought it out at the right time."

A year ago, Bubbles told me something similar at Fairfield:

"It sounds like I came around at the right time in your life," she'd said.

"But it could have happened earlier, too," Sam continued. "If you had a real good friend. Who was your best friend before Bubbles?"

I hesitated, my mind having drawn a blank.

"You see," he responded. "In my opinion, you didn't really have a significant good friend before Bubbles. What about a relative who you were close to?"

The question filled me with dread: The relative to whom I felt closest was my uncle, who'd physically abused me throughout my childhood, caused the leg injury that left me in pain and debilitated while I was working on the cancer vaccine, and amounted to nothing but a flatterer who stole essentially everything from me.

"So, until Bubbles, you didn't really understand a good personal relationship," he declared. "Because you didn't have one. But then, because of Bubbles, I think you found a relationship with sara - Because you were more receptive."

"You see, Pebbles opened up a door for you," he asserted. "It made you less fearful of having friends. It made you aware of what a better friend could be. All kinds of things like that."

"So, you were very fortunate to have run into her," he concluded…

I commented that when I left the relationship with Bubbles to continue my college research and pursuit of the cancer vaccine, she expressed understanding, saying, "Michael, I don't want to change that. I've always admired that about you. I wish I could sit down and study like you…"

And I was going to honor her belief in me. As such, nothing was going to stop me until I had achieved that goal - I had to honor that sacrifice.

"Right," Sam said. "I can see that. I think she made you independent because of the way you parted. You were not afraid to go on your own. And what you thought to do was a good choice, because it gave you confidence."

"It all makes sense," he concluded. "It's not rocket science. It's just like they say: A person can set you on the right path in your life. That's why a lot of people will say, 'It was this teacher that really got me going', or, 'It was some acquaintance that really got me going.' Everybody needs a North Star in your life. It just shows you how influential people can be in both good and bad ways…"

It struck me that I had not responded to his question about a good friend before Bubbles by telling him about Reuben? Reuben had taken the path of becoming a dancer, and was dancing in Reno while I was at UC Davis, so that I would go and enjoy his shows, and he lived the whole thing with pebbles with me.

Recently, I'd told him about my getting together with Bubbles for the day on July 5. And he responded like, "Mike, where she has opened the door to you to her life, aren't you going to follow your heart and be with her this time? Drop everything you're doing and take a job in Las Vegas?"

And I said, no, I'm going to Yale. My legacy is about the work I leave behind. If she wants to follow me to Yale, I wouldn't try to protect her from those aspects of my father in me. But I'm pursuing my work… What I was put in this world to do…

"Exactly," Sam responded. "The way I see it from everything that you've told me, I think you are very fortunate to have had pebbles in your life, but I don't see pebbles as someone in your future.

"You met, you came together, you crossed, and you traveled the same path for a while, and now you have to go back to your individual path and diverge, because being together would really make you not go down the path that you were meant to and would make you the most happiest, and would make her the most happiest, either."

Nodding, I knew he was right.

So, with that, I asked my friend how he was doing?

"I'm just resting," he said. "I feel weak. I'm just getting to the point that I'm going to just continue sliding down. I'm just trying to slow my descent down. That's all…"

"I keep expecting that if I rest, I will regain some strength and energy," Sam continued. "But that comes slower and slower, and takes longer and longer. And every time I finish my rest, and I do exert myself, I'm not as strong, and I'm weaker and continue to slide.

"But if I don't get that rest, then I'm in strain mode and that is very uncomfortable and painful.

"So, rest is important, but I've been feeling like I'm falling into longer and longer rest."

"I call it, 'Degradation'," Sam declared. "Because that's the way I consider it.

"Because in a normal life, we have what we need to make us able to move about and move forward.

"But in my case, the future is that I will pass away. So, it's just preparing my way for that point.

"And that's the way it's going to be. And even though I'm trying to fight it, I'm still going to die in the end."

"So, do you fight it?" he asked, rhetorically. "And how much do you fight it? The way I look at it, you can do things so that my breathing is better, and I should continue to do those things that helped me optimize my condition, rather than let it slip more quickly.

"So, I'm just doing as much as I can. When I feel up to it, I do as much of a workout as I can, though I try to limit it to what is comfortable.

"And I'll just continue to do that, because that's all I can do. If I try to push it any further, I think I will accelerate my degradation. Because I'm just wearing myself out and causing damage."

I thought about my long COVID folks with post exertional malaise, who get worse with exertion and exercise.

"But I am doing things that allow me to breathe better," he asserted, "like the nebulizer and the flutter valve and the percussion massager. I've been seeing them working, and I just gotta continue to do those things. Get on the OneWheel, maybe five or ten minutes at the most and allow my legs to work out a little bit."

He got off the table.

"Anyway, Mike, it's always good talking to you."

He indicated that it was going to be Harlow's that he took May to dinner for her birthday.

"May likes it," he said. "So that's her birthday present."

I closed up the massage table and put it to the side and left, so Sam could have some time to rest before he took his wife out for her birthday...

CHAPTER TWENTY-ONE

Monday, July 21, 2025

I told steve about the good response that Sam had to that very interesting treatment of competing forces, saying that afterwards he was able to have a nice dinner with his wife.

Still, I was worried his expected downward descent.

"So, it's impossible for him to connect with anything now?" Steve asked. "Because that sounds like what you're saying. And if he could connect with this energy through what you were doing, he could connect with an energy that could help him transition to whatever he's going to transition to. Because he could ride that energy. Actually, he could become that energy ultimately when his body goes.

"I mean, that's the way I see it. That's what I'm working towards. Hopefully not until I'm 100. But I'm working towards this thing where you become the energy of transition. So, as painful as it is, and as awful as it is… Well, I want lots of drugs if it's painful. That goes without saying. But being on this energy - Riding on this energy wave that here you are bringing the energy up and conveying energy to him and presenting at all, and he's saying, 'No, no, it's all painful.' So, I don't understand him? I don't understand why he's doing that? Because what would it hurt? It could do so much good to embrace the energy. So, what does it do for him not to embrace it? To poo poo it? You become the pain, instead of becoming the energy."

I said that he was thinking human being, who I have appreciated all these years for that thinking capacity, and he is capable of thoughts beyond treating this like an energy that can help.

"'Thinking'," Steve repeated. "You've just hit something there. It's all in nature. So, there's nothing supernatural here. There's nothing irrational here. The only irrational thing here is that he's in so much pain, when he's had such a wonderful intellectual life. And it's nothing that you can reason yourself out of. So, if he could be smart enough to realize that he can't reason himself through this, then just experience what's inside, and experience what's being offered to you.

"I mean, what's being offered to him is so much more than what's offered to most people, in terms of the bioenergy and the Qi Gong that you're doing on him. And I wish he could just say, 'OK, what can it possibly hurt to say everything is in nature, so I don't have to be irrational, I don't have to go against my mind. But just experience what's in nature? And this energy is in nature.'"

Well, look, he has no idea that the end can be depressing. He's having nightmares about seeing all these sorrowful souls, crowded together in a black-and-white awful place, where the energy of this world is sucked out of these poor souls. So, where he's going, he sees as a potentially really bad place. So, it's hard for him.

"I get that it's hard for him," Steve replied. "But if he's going to reason through it, it is so much better for him to be in positive energy, then to be a hungry ghost with a whole bunch of other hungry ghost. I mean, that certainly stuff that's in the liturgy of a lot of things and in the experience of a lot of people."

He described his mother's experience.

"She suffered from thoughts of all these hands grasping at her and trying to pull her in, and she was terrified of it," he said. "But with her dementia, that kind of stopped, and towards the end, she was singing songs from the time that she was in the Army - singing, 'Oh, how I hate to get up in the morning', and, 'I'm going to murder the bugler', and she would laugh and laugh and laugh when she'd sing these songs. So, I think she was in a better place when she did go - when she transitioned…"

Sara wondered if the reason that I was having these really different energy experiences with Sam - with competing energies, etc. - wasn't because he was terminally ill.

"When was the last time you worked with someone with terminal illness?" she asked.

I responded that it was about 25 years ago, when I worked with Angie, not long after ethel.

"Well, maybe now that you're a more developed energy healer, it makes sense that you'd have different experiences with someone with terminal illness," she said.

She added that I had followed Ini through her terminal illness process.

"And you are following Cat Chow," she added. "So, it's not totally true that you haven't been around the dying process. Maybe humans are just a little different? When you do the energetic healing with Ini and Cat Chow, does it feel different than with humans? Or the same?"

I didn't think it was as intense. Generally, the energy just flows. Certainly, I wasn't having any of these competing energy experiences with Ini and Cat Chow.

I added that I didn't remember having any energy experiences with Ini while she was suffering with cancer, outside of those that drove me to bringing her to the emergency room at UC Davis.

"After Ini died, you had them," sara said.

Yes, for sure.

"Did you do any bioenergy on her while we knew she had cancer?" Sara asked.

I didn't think so. I didn't remember. All I remembered was trying to help her to eat by cooking for her, and getting help from others to apply those fentanyl patches.

I guess when we got that cancer diagnosis for her, I just thought it was over. and it was just applying those fentanyl patches and trying to get her to eat.

The night before on Saturday while we were at Karaoke, sara indicated that she needed to leave because she was having flashbacks about that time.

"I don't even know why my mind went to Ini?" she said. "I don't focus on her on a daily basis anymore - Thank God. But I had a flashback to the look she gave us right before she died, and I needed a little bit of time to decompress after that."

At the time, that was a very hard moment for me, too. Later, I treated it as Ini's greatest moment - When she fought to be with us in spite of all that suffering...

CHAPTER TWENTY-TWO

Wednesday, July 23, 2025

Sam joined the Qi Gong group long enough to tell us that he was feeling too fatigued to perform the self-practice with us before making a hasty retreat.

"How is Sam?" Ruth asked.

I described our recent conversations, and Sam's referring to his illness like a wound that doesn't heal.

I also commented that Sam was uncomfortable with Jeff making him the focus of the sessions.

"I'm sorry that Sam had such a negative response," ruth said. "He must've been listening. I wasn't."

Yes, Sam said that he was concerned that his tendency to care was getting in the way of his healing. To the point that he was telling me not to share as much.

"I just read something about empaths," Ruth said. "Becoming an empath is also a trauma response. Empaths have to learn how to be more selective they get with people, because with some people, it's not helpful for them to try to help."

I thought Sam could go into an unhelpful loop when it comes to the negativity of the world. He tries to figure out these difficult questions of why things are happening in the world, and I regard them as impossible to figure out because it's so irrational. Yet he gets stuck there, and I feel like it's been a difficult path in this life for him as a result.

Ruth commented that it sounded like Sam was ruminating on things that were better let go.

"And it's very draining," she said.

Ruth commented that a reason why it was hard on Sam to deal with insensitive people was because he could sense that, too.

It had been my general observation with Sam that he was very giving with people who I regarded that way. As for me, I would not enter into relationships with folks like those, because I wanted relationships that offered an equal exchange, and if I was with someone where it felt like I was just going to be giving and they weren't going to be giving back, then I quickly sized that person up and decided this wasn't someone with whom I wanted a relationship.

However, Sam had commented that he was disappointed in the way of the world and people not having integrity like they used to.

"So, he needs to come to terms that he has to protect himself somewhat," ruth said. "Because he gives so much that it's taking away his energy now. And he needs to restore that energy for himself.

"I think it's like when I had breast cancer: I was told that I need to do everything I can to take care of myself to strengthen my immune system and let everything else go.

Rosa commented that she had to do the same thing when it came to her Covid.

"Before, I was very, very active, and I just had to let everything go, "Rosa said. "And that was very hard for me because I have a type a personality, but I really need to do that for my healing.

"Some people can really drain you of energy," Rosa added. "If I'm in a good place, I can handle it. But if I'm not, and I'm feeling like I don't have that energy for myself, I can't deal with someone else who drains my energy."

I thought that Sam could do to rejuvenate himself was give of his wisdom to those who appreciate it. I felt like it was a very important meaningful act whenever he shared his wisdom with me, and a lot more important than making his bed or doing the dishes.

Indeed, on one occasion, Sam had told me, "If you're not able to give back to someone… Well, what good are you?"

"Yes," ruth said. "It sounds like it's hard for him to know when to give and when not to give. And that's something that he's going through right now. He has to realize that he has is a gift, and it would be nice if he could give it to everyone, and he has for years, but now it's time for him to be more selective."

"Yeah," Rosa added. "It's all about pacing"

"Because now when he's giving," Ruth inserted, "he's giving from his own energy source, and he needs that energy source for himself.

I asked ruth to clarify her comment.

"You mentioned that Sam, giving of himself is his gift, but it also gives him energy," she responded. "But it just has to be given and received as you would. If he just gives it and it falls on death ears, then he's giving away his wisdom, his energy, his strength when he needs it himself."

Ruth went on and said that she felt we all have certain gifts, and again it was just that, at times, we need to be selective about who we give that to so that we can maintain our own energy.

"It's like the story of us all having a bucket of stuff that we can share with people," she said. "But to replenish that bucket, we need to get it back. And if we just keep on giving it and giving it, our bucket becomes empty, and then we have nothing left to give even to ourselves."

Rosa commented that she had to make such adjustments herself, saying that she did not have the same energy level as she did before contracting Covid.

"Whereas my husband still does," she continued. "He still has his energy level. And we have an agreement that there are certain times when I just have to say, 'Not right now. I need my space. I need my time.' And it has nothing to do with him. It's just me needing to go back to my cocoon and try to re-energize myself. I don't need him for that, and I just need to do that within myself. And he respects that and it makes it so much better for both of us…"

I decided to call Sam and ask if he'd like to join us for the self-practice portion of the virtual group meeting?

Sam again indicated that he was feeling tired.

"I started by feeling well, but it seems like I've gone downhill," he said. "So, I don't know if it would be the best thing to do to listen to you."

Ruth and Rosa sent Sam their best wishes.

"You're always in our thoughts," ruth said. "We'll send you healing energy and love."

"Yep," Rosa added. "Take care of yourself. That's the right thing to do."

Initiating the self-practice, I found that the energy was bringing my hands just some 2 inches apart, so that they were a lot closer than usual. In addition, I was feeling some heat in my hands as opposed to the usual breeze?

And when my hands finally went about arching apart, it was excruciatingly slowly, is though being pushed out by these tiny waves extending perhaps a millimeter at a time.

Ruth commented that she was feeling swirling energy and her arms were going in circles, and this reminded me about the experience that I had with Sam on Sunday, such that I felt this competing energy coming out at me out of nowhere, even though I was already plugged into his energy body.

"They just blew at me from nowhere," I said.

Even when my hands finally are apart, to move them upwards was excruciatingly slowly again.

As it was, I was already feeling significant energy at my upper third eye and crown chakra, so I didn't know that was all that necessary for me to lift my hands all that much?

"Yeah, to get out of your head and into your heart and balance the two," ruth commented.

Rosa commented that as well as heart, Sam had this great intellect, so he had the two.

"It seems like great generous people are drawn and attracted to Qi Gong," ruth said.

Rosa commented that she had a very interesting energy experience.

"While you were talking, I felt a great big break, so that I felt like I was holding a pulsating beach ball, and it just kept rising and rising, and rising, and when it got up to my head, and my third eye, it was a brilliant white that I saw," she said. "My eyes were closed the whole time, but I'm seeing a brilliant white. And I'm perspiring like crazy, and I don't normally perspire. So, there's a lot of movement going on, and then all the sudden it just kind of released, and then I felt calm and just felt like I was coming back down to earth."

"I've never had that kind of sensation," she continued. "It felt like a beach ball, pulsating back-and-forth. Pretty exciting."

I was reminded of my first intimate experience with Elizabeth ("guru" from my years in DC) where there was this sheen that seemed like the manifestation of turbid Qi that exuded from her pores; and I felt happy that maybe she was undergoing some cleansing and getting all this "bad stuff" out.

"I usually don't perspire, but many times coming out of our sessions, my under arms are wet," Rosa admitted. "I have to go home and shower."

"Kind of like my own sweat lodge," Rosa concluded…

After the self-practice, I told Sara that I was pained about Sam.

She thought it was perhaps related to the feelings of guilty I still hold for my mother?

And yes, I still blame myself that she died alone, and now I feel so bad that Sam's dying.

And I have all this training in Qi Gong and energy medicine, and I believe it can make a difference, but the reality is, it's not.

"You're not God," Sara responded...

CHAPTER TWENTY-THREE

Saturday, July 22, 2025

I called Sam and asked if I could be of help?

"So nice of you to offer your time," he responded. "My daughter and grandson are coming today, and so I'll be spending time with them. I'm sorry that I haven't reached out to you. It's just that these days, I've just been focused on hour to hour. So, it's taking up my time - When things get down to minute to minute, that's when things really fall off."

I told him I just wanted him to know that I was out there, and if I thought I could help, then I wanted to.

"Oh, I really, really appreciate that," he replied. "It's nice to have that kind of support."

He talked about going to the doctor yesterday because he was experiencing numbness in his left arm and leg.

"They're going to give me an MRI on my back and head," he said. "So, they just want to check it out and see if there's anything going on there with the nerves and brain."

Sounded pretty brainless on their part, I thought, sarcastically. What a waste of time - Especially for a man who's breathing was labored and coughing increased. How is he going to tolerate an MRI? How much would that take out of him?

"There's always something that's gonna keep popping up," Sam continued. "Seems like you try to improve on one thing, and you might get a little bit better for whatever you're trying to improve, but then something else seems to go out," he said. "So, it's just one of those things, where it kind of seems like Whac-A-Mole."

At least he hadn't lost his humor and gift for metaphors, I thought.

"Anyway, I've got a prepare for my daughter coming over, so I'm going to get back to that," he said. "I hope that's something exciting happens to you."

I told him that I was planning on singing "Crazy Train" in memory of the lovable Prince of Darkness, Ozzy Osbourne, one of sara's favorite heavy metal singers.

Sam shared his wealth of knowledge about Ozzy Osbourne, starting with Black Sabbath. I told him about the concert that Osbourne performed two weeks ago, which had Sara transfixed while watching online, throwing her head back-and-forth, her hair flying, as this usual flower girl transformed to a heavy metal girl.

"Enjoy your tribute to Oz," he said, concluding the call…

CHAPTER TWENTY-FOUR

Wednesday, July 30, 2025

Sam joined us for the virtual Qi Gong meeting, saying that he was feeling well at the moment.

Ruth complained that she had been feeling an unusual amount of fatigue during the week.

Sam wondered if it wasn't because of the warmer weather?

Ruth then shared that last week, her cat, Chloe, shot right in between her legs while she was doing the Qi Gong self-practice and that was unusual because her cat was blind.

"It's interesting that when you're doing Qi Gong, you wonder, 'Is it something internal? Or is it something outside?'" Sam speculated.

"Exactly," ruth said. "And she's blind. I don't know how she got between my legs without even touching. I just felt her go through. Because, otherwise, she does bump into things. I mean, my legs were not open that wide, and she went right between them. So maybe she could sense the Qi, so she could walk right through them?"

Of late, I'd become interested in echolocation as performed by bats and other species, so to lead me to wonder if the energy of Qi Gong can be sensed by animals?

Furthermore, I was wondering if a perception of Qi can facilitate an integration and understanding of the size and location of something?

"I think when you are in a nice, neutral state, you are able to sense things," Sam asserted. "You know, we do have our senses, and they do seem to be heightened when we allow ourselves to be open to

them. So, that might be a big part of it - That you're quite open to feeling anything that activates your senses…"

Initiating the Qi Gong self-practice, I immediately perceived a tingling energy all around my fingers, which was not the way I usually experience the energy between my hands.

My hands moved apart, but like last time, they did so exceedingly slowly; and also, in waves, so that there was this wave of energy producing a slight motion at the hands, which was also different from anything I'd experienced before in the self-practice.

I was already feeling energy at the top of my head - This before I felt any energy leading my hands to go upwards; and when they did move upwards, my hands did something of a little game of twister, which was also unusual...

As the energy left my hands to signal the end of my self-practice, I invited the others to comment about their experience?

Ruth talked about feeling the energy in her head in a way that she hadn't experienced before.

"I feel it come out of one of the chakras at my head," she said. "But this time I feel it like it's energizing me from inside my head."

"It's interesting for me," Sam began, "because I'm doing it outside, and it starts with the hands, but it seems like my arms and my face and such, and because I'm outdoors, I can feel the breeze, and it just seems very relaxing. Calming - From my hands to the rest of my body.

"And it's just a nice feeling. You just feel like you're part of the rest of the world. You don't just feel anything energetic that's just within you, but everything around you feels very connected."

This was the highlight of the evening: Sam had basically energetically melted into everything around him, which was what I wished for him when it came to his passing/transitioning.

Ruth commented that she had a similar feeling when she did Qi Gong.

"Because when I do the self-practice, and even when Dr. Mike would be doing the practice on us individually, I would feel a certain happiness," she said. "Joy. And it's not connected with anything in particular. It's just I'm happy. I'm feeling joy."

Sara had been in the room with me, performing the self-practice, and I asked if she was experiencing anything?

She commented that she was feeling relaxed.

Next to me, was our cat, which was laying down with her open belly, signaling that she was relaxed, as well.

"I imagine that an animal feels very calm in their surroundings when their surroundings are calm," Sam commented. "So, I think that animals perceive their surroundings very well, just like humans. So, it doesn't surprise me that if you're relaxed, Mike, the cat would be relaxed, as well…"

CHAPTER TWENTY-FIVE

Sunday, August 3, 2025.

Talking with my friend Reuben, I shared my feelings of guilt where Sam was concerned, saying that since I'd known Sam, he had this odd constellation of symptoms, from skin eruptions to chronic cough (that even he felt were psychosomatic!), but now I felt I hadn't acted on them enough.

"You recommended to him that he get diagnosed," Reuben responded, matter of factly.

Yes, but, in retrospect, he was less than diligent; and I kept doing the Qi Gong treatments anyway, despite him fudging along and making excuses about not liking this doctor and that one, and believing what he was telling me; namely, that this was a mental thing and he just had to deal with it on his own, and he knew what the problem was, blah blah blah.

"But did he want those or believe in those treatments?" Reuben asked.

Perhaps not, but I should have pushed harder? I should have told him, "Sam, I'm not working with you until you've been evaluated by the medical community to my satisfaction"?

Especially since he was literally the one who came up with the Qi Gong corollary that people need to be thoroughly medically evaluated before you do Qi Gong on them. Otherwise, there was the potential for delay of care.

So, it weighs on me.

Though, in truth, there have been many cases that I've had when I attempted bioenergy on someone who need conventional care, I'd get the shell effect; that is, the feeling like there was an energy shell around them, so that I wouldn't be able to perform bioenergy, and I'd tell the person you need to go to a doctor.

But was I blindsided in this case? Because of my emotional ties, or what this person could give me, so that I kept working on him anyways?

"I don't think you should second-guess yourself, " Reuben said. "If you helped him feel better, and if he wasn't going to go to those doctors anyways, why not help him?"

"And who's to say what they could've done?" he added. "Whether it would've been better?"

"And there's no saying that they could've done anything for him," he continued. "There's a lot of things that they truly can't do much for. And there are some where treatments have consequences where the treatment is worse than the disease.

"I mean, if it was me, I'd want to know everything there is to know first. That's why I call you. Because I know I get the most honest answers from you that you would know from the medical world. If I tried to talk to a regular doctor about that, they'd give me an abrupt answer and that would be it. They'd say, 'We can put you on this, or we can put you on that', and then they'll get annoyed with me if I ask them any questions, like, 'How did the medicines work? And are there non-medicine options?'

"And that's the difference: You are not offended by me asking you questions about going on medications. You're someone who would respect it. You're an open person who strives to find the truth in things. You understand enough to know that doctors don't know everything. They might be able to give you a better answer than a layman, but most people in the medical field now, they get so bent out of shape if you don't do what they tell you to do, or if you question them…"

Reuben related Sam's condition to having cancer.

"And what do you do for cancer?" he asked, rhetorically.

You cut it out, I responded. And then give them chemotherapy. That's pretty much what most doctors would do.

"Right," he responded. "But there's a lot of people out there that aren't about to go through that."

"My dad refused it," he continued. "He wasn't about to get cut open and then thrown on chemotherapy - even though that was what his doctors recommended treatment for it."

"And I doubt very much that I would," he added. "Maybe if I was young and had little ones ?" He said. "But being older and not

having little ones, I don't think I would go that route. For myself, I'd want other avenues…"

Later, Sam and I talked, and he told me about new difficulties when it came to eating, saying that food didn't taste good anymore.

"As soon as I touch what I eat, it just turns 'ugly'," he said. "I can't eat anything. So, I'm basically not eating anything hardly at all."

"I'm always weak," he continued. "I can't even do half my routine. Yesterday I felt a pain in my chest that was excruciating. It was sort of like a sampler of how it's going to be. It was very difficult. I think I'm getting so close to that threshold point, so that I'm dipping into it every once in a while and can barely pull myself out.

"I was laying there, resting before going to see my aunt and family at my sister's house, and all of a sudden, it just hit me in my chest. It felt like my chest collapsed down, and I said, 'OK, this might be it.'

"And then, I pulled out – Barely! But it's just like the slope of my decline has gone to a point where it's right at the threshold point. And now I keep slipping into that threshold area."

"So, I think that's what it's trying to tell me," he concluded…

I asked Sam to elaborate on what he experienced, so I could better understand it.

"It's kind of hard to describe," he began. "There was nausea and tightness, pressure, all kinds of things that just make you feel like you're helpless, but it has a ramification throughout the body, saying, 'OK, nothing can help you pull out of this area.'

"Like usually, when you feel something, your other system starts participating to try to help you. But there was no cavalry this time. There's something pulling me down. I don't know what it was? But it just sort of grabs you and releases you.

"Anyway, it's going to happen again, but it may not release me the next time. Or it may release me, but it's going to do further damage.

"Right now, I swear, I can't eat anything. Everything is hard to do. I try to get up, so that I can move about a bit, but then I have to go and sit down again.

"Anyway, it feels like all of this is sort of preparing me, and there's not much left to go on, and the alternative is much better…"

Then, Sam surprised me by saying he had plans to get a tooth extracted.

"I'm hoping that at least that will help with the headaches," he said. "And I'll get that done tomorrow - if I don't fall into a deep pit between now and then - and then maybe I could stop taking the Tylenol. But even then, it's just one more stone on the pile, so to speak."

I suggested he meet with palliative care and explained their purpose.

"Yes, that is somebody I do need to speak to, then," he said.

However, when we talked about the use of morphine in palliative care and hospice, he expressed reservations.

"I guess it makes it easier," he began. "I guess if you get the right dosage, you're still lucid enough and that may work.

"But right now, I'm not feeling pain; I'm just feeling real tired and weak. I have no energy. The real pain was what occurred yesterday for the first time. I guess if that pain comes back, and it persists, then I think there will be a need for palliative care - Definitely.

"But I'm not too sure, because that pain seems so excruciating. If that's going to be the nail that's driven into the coffin and there won't be much time after that.

"So, I'm just wondering if getting it will be helpful, because it will be too close to the end…"

I told Sam that palliative care and home hospice was about being able to cope with conditions like excruciating pain without going to the hospital.

"Yes, that would be good," he said. "Because I don't want to leave the house. Do I just call my doctor? I think it's time to throw the switch then."

Then, I asked if there was anything that I could do, like come over and perform Qi Gong?

"I would appreciate that," he said. "I'd hate to bother you, though."

It was no bother. It was the best use of my time that I could think of and asked if I could get him something at Ikeda's on the way?

"I can't think of anything, Mike," he said. "We have a lot of food. I just can't eat it. I wanted watermelon yesterday, and they got me watermelon. But as soon as I started eating it, it's really weird, Mike… All of these things that I like, all of a sudden, they taste, the best word is, 'ugly'. They taste really ugly or repulsive. It's amazing that feeling. I get nauseous. It's like my body is rejecting food. Even food that I used to really enjoy."

"All of my past comforts have been taken away," he declared. "I'm searching for some comfort, but, Mike, I can't find it."

"So, thank you Mike," he concluded, "but I think that I'm fine right now."

He was anything but 'fine right now', I thought.

I told him I would perform a review of the medical literature to understand his change in taste?

"Thank you, Mike," he responded. "Sometimes a simple answer is the best solution. But right now, it eludes me. Anyway, I look forward to seeing you. Bye-bye…"

I hurriedly got on the road: My driving seemed off, and I think because I was so upset.

Arriving at Sam's, I let him talk for a long time, because I thought (under the circumstances) it was important to listen as a friend.

He described the difference between purpose and passion.

"Purpose," he said, "was about performing a finite action. With passion, there's always more to it. You're never done exploring it. That's what I've been chasing - Is passion. All my life. In whatever I do. That's why I have all this stuff. Because I want to know more about it."

He talked about his Rubik's cube.

"I figured if I just kept learning about it and chipping away at it, I'd keep learning about it. And that's just like with everything I do. Baseball. Football. Skating. Whatever. I mean, who pursues skiing so much that they end up buying an endless slope and teaching it? Not very many people.

"This is why the process I'm going through is very intriguing. It's now becoming a passion. I'm finding out and thinking, 'OK, what's my next step?'

"But the problem with passion is that it blinds you. And sometimes you miss the obvious. Or you take a wrong path.

"That's the thing about passion: You take the wrong path, and you travel down that path, and then you realize you were on the wrong path. And you have to double back and take another path to find what you're looking for and get on the correct path. But for me, I think time is running short."

There was no question that time was running short, I thought.

"And the thing about passion, too, is sometimes you realize that you can be satisfied with moderation. But the thing about passion is, you're willing to pursue it, even if you don't get far with it."

"But sometimes it's really important work," he concluded, "and you'll leave the further finding of it to someone else…"

He returned to the topic of palliative care.

"Because I don't know what my course is that I'll be going to?" he said. "It may be tremendously painful - Tremendously so! And it will not be worth it to take on that pain. So, it would be good to be sedated at least through that course until I reach the point that it ends."

Earlier, Sam had talked about what it was to nearly drown and the struggle to breathe and the purgatory in between breaths.

I thought that opioids could reduce that time in purgatory, and that was usually the body's response to such a situation anyways; that is, releasing all kinds of endogenous opioids and endorphins when you get to that point, the body is going to put you in a suspended state of animation; namely, the freeze response. So, why not let medical science intervene in a humane way, instead of going through that purgatory?

I mean, as long as we knew the end was coming, why not just accept it? Why be put through this purgatory? Just permit someone to give you some morphine, instead of being put through all the suffering for no good reason?

"Sure," he said. "But just enough to take the edge off of it. Not overdo it…"

Sam talked about his planned tooth extraction and feeling fortunate that he had Dr. Kubota as a dentist.

"Because Dr. Kubota is very skillful."

He shared a story from years ago about being referred to an orthodontist.

"The orthodontist did a lot of work on me," Sam said. "But he didn't charge me for it, because I had helped him with skiing.

"But then he told me that I had to get out to an oral surgeon right away because the tooth had gone so bad.

"But when I told Dr. Kubota about what the oral surgeon had planned, he said, 'I'll do it.'

"And Dr. Kubota reminds me of my uncle. Because my uncle was very skilled like that. He was a great doctor. He wanted to be a surgeon, but he left surgery school so that he could help his brother-in-law, who had a practice and was getting up in age. So, he took over his practice. And he was so good. He was like an old-time doctor. He did surgeries. He did everything. He was just really good. And at his funeral, there were so many people. He was also President of the AMA. He was just remarkable. And Dr. Kubota reminds me of him.

"So, when Dr. Kubota said, 'No, I can do it', I trust him.

"And he's been great. He doesn't charge me hardly anything for his work, because he knows that I don't have insurance. He done things for me for free. Emergency visits. He just says, 'Don't worry about it.'

"So, what I'm trying to say is, man, I am so fortunate in this life. I mean, there's a lot of bad things - like these vents that they've screwed up. But that's minor, compared to the larger picture of things…"

Sam talked about hope.

"You're always wondering if something will break free and send this moving in the right direction, rather than the negative direction?" he began. "Maybe my fibrosis is at a point that it's improving, so that the adhesions will start to decrease and become better? I mean, there are certain signs like my breathing has improved. And I didn't think that would happen - Inhaling and taking my breaths - Breathing out slowly. It was so hard in the beginning. Now it has improved. I feel like I'm inhaling better, especially with the help of the nebulizer. But yet, everything seems to keep declining. So, it's these weird positive things I get that keep me wondering? I mean, I can still sit up. I can sit down. I can still balance. But I wonder when that's gonna go away, too?"

He suggested we do Qi Gong.

"What do you think?" he asked. "Do you think some external Qi Gong will be of aid to me right now?"

I thought it was worth a try.

From the beginning, it was an interesting experience: The energy directed my hand like the wing of a plane, and I was feeling the energy blowing out of Sam's chest like it was running over both sides of my hand like the picture of what gives a plane lift.

And then it took my hand closer to Sam, despite that interesting feeling.

Sam wondered if I might be feeling his breath as he coughed?

No, not a chance, I responded. This was energy…

As I performed external Qi Gong, Sam talked about the MRI he had earlier in the day.

I listened in disgust.

So stupid, I thought. A fella unable to breathe complains of hand tingling – because he has no oxygen in his system! – and they're putting through an MRI. What a waste of time for a man who has no time! Fucking stupid doctors. What the hell are they thinking?...

The energy took me a good distance away from Sam ultimately to the other side of the room.

Then, the energy left my hands, so that I was effectively done

"Good," Sam declared. "Thank you, Mike. It feels like I'm done, too."

I froze, fearing the implications of what his saying "done" meant.

Fortunately, this was not the case.

"Today I feel like you did something," he continued. "I can't tell you what. But right now, I sure do feel different than I did before. I feel a bit more energetic. Like my head is buzzing, but evenly throughout my whole skull. It's very slight, but you can feel it still. And you've helped me breathe better. My chest is lighter. I think you've done something Mike. More than before. Either that, or I'm a more sensitive to it. My chest feels more expensive. Like it's expanding. And my head feels like it's a little bit lighter. And overall I feel much better. Thank you. it's good. I felt this more than I have in the past. I think the worse I get, the more I'll be able to feel it."

"In fact," he concluded, "it makes me feel like eating a chocolate."

And with that, he invited me to share some chocolate with him...

Entering the dining room, Sam pointed to the windows and described how earlier in the day, his brother, Stanley, had asked what he could do to help?

"I said I'd like to be able to look through the windows in the kitchen nook," Sam recounted, "because I was spending a lot of time there."

Yeah, trying to eat through everything tasting 'ugly', I thought.

"So, Stan cleaned the windows," he declared.

Listening, I recalled what Elizabeth told me when I'd gone to help Bubbles' mother thirty years ago:

"You've captured the essence of what love is all about. It has to do with little things, like compassion and respect, concern and attentiveness..."

Making my way to the door, Sam said that the one thing he was going to miss was getting reports from me from Yale about how well I was doing.

"I know you're going to do really well there," he said.

I was deeply touched.

Then, he thanked me for being such a good friend and coming to help…

Driving away, though, I couldn't help but think of some of the things he told me:

"It feels like climbing your way through the desert before you get to the oasis."

But given his condition, it seemed his situation was more like clawing your way through the desert till you get to the mirage!

I was losing hope. It seemed to me he was indeed "degrading", and rather than a lot of agony, I'd like to see him be able to sidestep all that and take advantage of modern medicine delivering exogenous endorphins (namely, opioids) and peacefully taking that path into the great beyond…

Sara also commented about all the stupid things that the medical system was putting Sam through.

"They put him through a sleep study," she began. "What were they going to do? Put him on CPAP? People have a real hard time with that. Like why would they make his life difficult, trying to get adjusted to CPAP? Why were they taking an MRI of his spine? What? Are you going to do surgery? Like who's gonna do surgery on someone like that? He's going to die on the table! Like, what are you thinking? What the hell? At this point in the game, you would think that you would only want to do things that would result in actionable treatment that will improve his quality of life; and anything that will cause suffering or it's just academic and about knowing something or long-term, chronic management… Well, he's just past the point of that."

"If it's something that they can do to make him more comfortable, then go ahead," she concluded. "That can make him less anxious - That can help him adjust to being so short of breath - Please help him with that - Those compassionate things to make him feel comfortable...

CHAPTER TWENTY-SIX

Wednesday, August 6, 2025

Sam asked me to call him during my lunch break: He sounded weak and breathless, like he was really struggling, and talked about difficulty laying down and getting up, saying that he was feeling queasy.

"I'm feeling more tired all the time," he said. "And when I get up, I lose all appetite," he said. "I was wondering if you had any thoughts on that?"

With all the nausea and loss of appetite and things tasting bad, I could easily imagine him getting dehydration and suggested drinking as much as he could.

He responded that that would be difficult because he was going for a sleep study tonight.

What was the sleep study for? I thought. Would it help him with a terminal lung condition? Or was it another stupid test (like the MRI) to figure out another relatively meaningless symptom in a man who was dying?

"It seems that now any testing is pointless," Sam added.

Then, Sam told me that some doctor looked at the MRI result and because there was a comment about a minimal compression at the cervical spine, sent him to the emergency room yesterday.

"The conclusion was, it's there," he said. "I have it. But it's not to the point that it's causing any major issues"

Duh! Like there was ever any emergency? It just seemed like a lot of Ooga Booga they were putting this poor man through!

"Oh, everything is taxing right now," Sam said.

And the medical system was just adding to that.

Meanwhile, Sam was still having headaches, though it moved from one side to the other, so we went back to the dentist, who examined him and didn't find any more cavities, but thought he was dealing with a sinus infection.

"It's amazing how when you worry, your worry makes the injuries happen," he said. "But it sure is draining. I wish I was in better shape through all this. Going through this is very taxing now. I tell you, walking is getting more and more difficult."

He sounded so weak and alone. It just sounded like he was being tortured.

"Now, it's just a matter of living by inches at a time," he said. "But those inches go a long way."

I want to ask him if he'd reached out to palliative care but didn't have the heart.

I wished him a good sleep study and told him we'd be thinking about him during the Qi Gong self-practice.

"Thank you, appreciate that," he responded. "I'm sure I'll feel all of you. Just wish me for a good night's sleep. Take care. Bye-bye."

Ending the call, it struck me that today was Hiroshima Day, where's Sam's family originated and had been bombed to smithereens...

CHAPTER TWENTY-SEVEN

Friday, August 8, 2025

Sam was not at all well when I called him.

"The pain of living is worse than dying," he said. "I just don't think it's worth it anymore."

Then, he thanked me for calling and hurriedly got off the phone...

CHAPTER TWENTY-EIGHT

Saturday, August 9, 2025

During the night, an ambulance had to be called to rush Sam to the Emergency room.

"Mike, I was so out of it," Sam began, breathlessly describing the ordeal. "I was just like Jell-O. I had no strength. I couldn't help them. I couldn't control my body. All I felt was people tugging on me. And I couldn't get air. I couldn't."

"It seemed like there were an army of people there at the house," he continued. "I asked May, and she said, 'Yeah, the bedroom was just packed with people.'"

"So, how was your work?" he asked.

I should have told him not to think about that now; but I decided to play it cool and go along and told him about the presentation I'd seen the other day about functional neurologic disorders, which encompasses neurologic conditions in which the patients suffered from neurologic symptoms that could not be explained by anything found on Neuroimaging or brain scans, so to suggest something wrong with the "software" of the brain. And listening, it was like a light went off in my head.

This is what happened to Kino, I thought. This is what external Qi Gong treats.

"That's really good," Sam commented. "You can relate to Qi Gong. I think Qi Gong is a way to fix the software glitches."

Yes, that was even the term the presenter used to describe the problem - "glitches."

So, even being near death and in utter extremis and fighting for his life, Sam was still capable of this kind of thought and able to perfectly grasp the implications and applications of what I was doing and put them perfectly into words. What in the world was I going to do without him?!

"And it has lots of uses," he continued. "I believe that…"

Sam talked about feeling bad about leaving others with a lot of tasks that he'd left undone.

"I feel like I'm washing my hands of it," he said. "And I feel so bad about that. And I think, 'If my death is really painful, then I can be more at peace with this.'"

One good thing about "slow and painful", I thought. Less guilt…

"So, have you heard from Yale?" Sam asked.

Yes, the credentialing process was moving forward.

"Are you finding it exciting?" he asked.

At times, yes, I said. At other times, with the weather being so nice and all the fruits on the trees, I think I'm going to miss leaving here.

Then, I stopped cold.

"Mike!" I thought. "Who do you think you're talking to?!"

"What is your top memory from your time in Sacramento?" he asked.

The first thought that popped into my head was one of our first days here when Sara, Ini and I were taking a walk along the river, and Sara made the sign of a heart with her hands as I photographed her.

"Good memory," he responded. "Have you spoken with Deane lately?... I think the cannabis helped a little bit. It didn't help enough, though. But a lot of it is psychological. I keep on looking for a way to relax, but the deeper I look, the more I get away from it."

Given that I start panicking upon experiencing the least bit of air hunger, I couldn't imagine what he was going through...

I asked if I could perform external Qi Gong? Then, connecting energetically, I perceived a feeling energy at his chest: It felt like energy blowing all around my hand and coming outward from his chest and, at the same time, pulling me towards him.

How does energy that feels like it's blowing at you pull your hand towards someone? I thought. Towards the source? Towards the person?"

I experienced a feeling of activation of my solar plexus? Then, it felt like my hand was energetically interacting with my Dantien, which I'd associate with my mother since the experience with her at the mortuary.

Was my mother somehow with us? I thought. Was she helping Sam crossover?

"You know, I was wondering if I would do anything differently?" he began. "Even all the bad things I did? All the things that I didn't like to do? That were too difficult, but I had to go through it anyway? But I wouldn't change anything. I've learned from everything. Even the most difficult things. If I had the power to change anything, I wouldn't. Because had I, I might not be in the position that I was in now."

Are you kidding? I thought. Who in the world would want to be in the position that he was in now?

"And even though it's a difficult space right now," he added. "I believe it's the right place to be in."

Jesus! I thought, disbelieving.

He said that if he had one wish, it was to still be able to give something while he was still here.

"It's like, over the past months," he began, "I've been meeting people, and they've been telling me about things that I don't remember. It's like I impacted their lives. And if I hadn't, they would have felt so much differently. So, I guess I don't have to worry about leaving something behind? Maybe I've already done that?"

"It's better to leave things behind as you travel, then dump it at the end of your destination," he advised. "It doesn't benefit very many people when you carry everything to the end. You should be parceling it out all along.

"I suppose this is my way of trying to say, 'Don't worry about the future. Don't worry about any other commitments. Just enjoy what you have.'"

He broke off.

"It's good to leave with a clear conscience," he concluded. "I didn't get it 100% every time, but if I got it 80%, it was good enough..."

"It will be neat when you go to the East Coast and start this new chapter in your life," Sam said. "It will be fun. A whole New World. Just like landing on a different planet almost when you go east. You're not going to recognize the landscape. But you'll adapt to it."

I was quiet. I didn't feel like I was going anywhere new. I'd lived in Connecticut. I'd experience the East Coast.

"So, what type of new lifestyle will you set for yourself and sara when you move back east?" he asked. "Do you have any plans for doing something more or less than you have been doing? Getting into something a little bit more deeply? Music? Plays?"

My thoughts were mainly on working.

"Yeah, but you have to make time for yourself," he responded. "Otherwise, you'll miss a lot. You'll be doing Qi Gong so much that you'll enjoy that, too. But don't forget about doing other things…"

Sam described the pain in his chest.

"It's stabbing," he said. "This pain just makes my whole upper body experience nauseousness and a feeling like, 'There's nothing you can do about it.' It's just very uncomfortable. It's like the worst discomfort you can get before it surges into pain. And I'd rather have the pain than this feeling, because it's so like I wish I die and it would be all over. I wish I could describe it better. Just this feeling in my lungs… It's rotating and it's so uncomfortable. I tried to stay away from it, but it just comes back."

I asked if I could check him energetically to try to understand the source of his pain?

"It's part of the pleural cavity," he asserted. "The lungs. It's like this thing growing throughout my body, and it's holding my chest in place. The sad thing is, it's got so embedded that it's permanent and it's continuing to take up real estate."

Connecting with him energetically, it like the energy from his chest was moving across my hand and into my dantian.

"What is my blood pressure?" he asked.

Looking at the monitor, it was 136/89.

"That's better than before," he said. "You're relaxing me..."

Sam described his as a "wonderful life."

"I mean, in terms of meeting wonderful people," he began, "and not meeting bad people... Well, that's how it was so wonderful.

"It sure was fun meeting you, Mike. At the roller rink. That's so funny. When I saw you, I just knew. I thought, 'I think this guy is going to be a cool guy to know.'

"All the times that we've discussed things and talked about bioenergy. It came at a good time in my life…"

I told Sam that I'd gone to Yoselin yesterday and considered giving her the book that I'd written about her. Reading through the book, Sam was in at least half of it, which I considered the better part of the book.

"Was it a pretty good story?" he asked. "Do you think the story is over with? Probably not."

I said that one thing was for sure - That woman sure did have an interesting healing effect on me.

Last night while Sam was fighting for his life, I was experiencing muscular releases in my hip at the very site of where I'd been injured by my uncle and that sent me on my bioenergy and Qi Gong journey; and it was also this place in my body that I could never get out on my own.

"It's amazing how we have little places that are known points with significant capability to produce symptomatology, and yet they're so tiny and so overlooked that their bypassed," he responded. "Until something points us in the right direction."

"And that's good that you found help with Jasmine," he added. "You're fortunate that you've actually found a guidepost. A lot of people actually don't find the right guidepost."

His comment led me to think about my brother, and what Cynthia had said of him: That he was just out there in the waves of the ocean, never finding his way...

Sam was aware that I'd had plan today to be on the road to help my father.

"I feel so bad that I robbed time from your dad and stepmother," Sam said.

I told him I wasn't and there was no more important place for me to be right now.

"Everything is turning against me," he said. "It's sort of like 'Last man standing.' That's what all my organ systems are playing. They're saying, 'We're gonna show you that we're still hardy.' And I'm like, 'You gotta let me go, because the big guy's just dead."

Just then, a medical resident came into the room and abruptly told Sam that he had hours today is to live, and so that his suffering wouldn't be prolonged, she had stopped his antibiotics, respiratory treatments and IV fluids.

"What?!" I said, aghast. "You don't have near enough information yet to make those kinds of declarations and decisions."

I insisted on speaking with her attending, and in the meanwhile, she immediately reactivate Sam's treatments.

The resident beat a hasty retreat, and I told Sam to have heart, and we'd navigate our way through this.

But Sam responded that it was OK, and he was not unhappy about those declarations.

"They're giving me the soft landing I've been looking for," he said...

"It's good that you stayed," Sara commented. "If you hadn't, Sam might have died of sepsis."

Yes, hopefully the medical establishment could afford him a "softer landing" than overwhelming infection by withholding treatment.

"So, everybody is in agreement that Sam doesn't have long to live, right?" she asked.

No, they weren't, I said. Talking with the Pulmonary fellow, he said that Sam had hours to days to live *without antibiotics*; however, with them, it wasn't impossible that Sam could live for months...

Later, the medical resident returned – this time accompanied by her attending.

The family offered their goals, saying that it was very important to them that Sam have a chance to recover from the present infection and that they were very thankful for my help and raising concern that Sam was not being treated with antibiotics on the ward.

"Sam has lots of family and friends," May said. "So, we want Sam to be able to say any goodbyes for maybe a week or two."

Sam said that he wanted to go home and was interested in hospice.

"Well, given your current oxygen requirement, we can send you home," the attending responded. "But hospice does not offer measures like oxygen, so, if you were to go home, it would be without oxygen."

Hearing this, my jaw dropped.

How in the world does that go along with any of the family or Sam's patient goals or requests? I thought. It's like she'd told them, "If you wanna die at home, we will help you, but it means that you die by suffocation." In general, everything that came out of this woman's mouth was so unkind and devoid of any semblance of human feeling.

Nevertheless, May continued in a poised, mature, polite manner, so I decide to stay in the background and, for the time being, treat this like mostly a family matter.

Finally, Sam declared that he wanted me to share his goals because he felt I could do it in a succinct way.

As it happened, I'd previously summarized those goals on the room's whiteboard and briefly commented on the different points:

1. *Palliative Care and Hospice referrals to assist in making informed decisions about end of life matters and attend Sam's suffering;*

2. Pulmonary input, regarding Sam's pneumonia, oxygen demand, chest discomfort due to the interstitial lung disease?
3. Mental health referral to evaluate for Sam's PTSD-related drowning trauma, which was being reactivated by his present shortness of breath;
4. Dietitian consult, especially regarding the problem that nothing tastes good to Sam anymore and his caloric intake was low.

And after listening to all of this, the resident and attending responded by staring blankly and saying nothing…

"Why are they so bad?" Sara asked of the resident and attending.

I didn't know. Indeed, a nurse who had been present in the room whispered to me, "Keep advocating", as though he knew something about how dense and unfeeling and unhearing and unreachable these doctors were.

"Will he possibly have a different attending tomorrow?" Sara asked.

No, Sam and the family indicated that were okay with working with them.

In addition, the family surprised Sam by telling him that his brother and sister were bringing his mother to see him, so that Sam teared up and became emotional like I'd never seen him.

The day before, when Sam and I were in the emergency room, he told me that something that saddened him was that he wanted to talk with his mother for one last time, but didn't think that he would be able to in his current state and indicated that he was just going to have to pass away without seeing or talking with her again.

Now, with the news that his mother was coming, I asked Sam if he was OK?

He responded that it was what it was, and he was just going to have to roll with it.

"My mom is a very strong person who's been through a lot," he said, "so I believe that she can get through this…"

"What are your plans for the rest of the day?" Sara asked.

I said I felt like Sam's condition was stable for now, and I still wanted to check on my father.

Before leaving the hospital, I put together that the cousin's (John) father was the uncle who Sam admired so much as a doctor and been such an important part of Sam's upbringing.

When I approach John and confided this to him, he responded by saying that he wished he had a few more hours with his father.

This had the effect of solidifying my feeling like I should spend some more time with my dad, and decided that as long as things were in a holding pattern here, I'd give Sam this time to privately be with his family and go visit my father...

CHAPTER TWENTY-NINE

Sunday, August 10, 2025

At my father's, I had a moment of weakness when I was in my father's work room, and looking at all of those tools and wrenches, and knowing that he could previously fix anything, and there I was so inept. And now his cognition was such that he'd never be able to show me how to use any of them…

Then, going into the house, I was surprised to have a very coherent conversation with father about Sam and way he was treated by the medical team in the hospital.

"That's crazy!" my father responded. "Really it is. Besides being dangerous."

He laughed, nervously.

"Oh, poor guy," he continued. "How is he doing now?"

I said Sam was doing better, and there were plans for palliative care to meet with him tomorrow.

"At least he has an advocate," my father said. "In you."

He shook his head.

"How did the doctors pass that off?" he asked, disbelieving that they would withhold care. "I really don't understand it."

Yes, it's just all struck me how much power doctors have. We could literally be the "high executioner" if we chose to.

"That's scary," he concluded. "It's just plain, outright scary… I don't know. You just don't know what you're getting into?…"

CHAPTER THIRTY

Tuesday, August 12, 2025

Arriving at the hospital after work at about 7 PM, I casually strode through the hallways to Sam's room. Over the past days, Sam had told me that he was no long requiring a high flow oxygen mask (delivering oxygen at a rate of 43 L per minute) and was doing well on oxygen via nasal cannula (at 2 L per minute). Hence, I was expecting to find his condition significantly improved.

What I found, instead, was my friend still shaken from something that happened to him a couple hours before.

In brief, he'd had an "attack" while in the bathroom, such that his oxygen levels dropped into the 30's. That was at 5PM. Now, it was 7PM, and he was still shaking.

"Mike, I can't go through that again," Sam told me, terrified. "And these guys are pushing me to go home. Every day they're saying, 'Sam, we have to talk about discharge. We have to make plans for you to go home.' And Mike, if I was at home, and what happened to me in that bathroom happened to me at home…"

He broke off and shook his head in complete and utter frustration.

"All I can do is suffer," he concluded. "Mike, how am I going to die?..."

"And why is that?" Sara asked of Sam's condition. "Because it's a terrible experience to go through? I mean, I don't have any experience with that."

Well, for we who do have experiences with air hunger, there's little worse: I know for me, when I experience air hunger, every second is a lifetime of unimaginable horror - I just experienced so much fright that I go insane.

And I can't even begin to imagine what Sam went through with an oxygen saturation in the thirties. And this happened in the auspices of a hospital, where they have every kind of assistance available to him for episodes like that - where he is surrounded by medical personnel. What are things going to be like when he is out of the hospital?

Sam said that he was being pressured by the medical team to make a decision about his discharge. But how can he or they fathom discharge of a patient like this when this is happening? How could they, in good faith, even suggest sending him home when this is happening right there in the hospital?

"And not only does he not want to leave the hospital now," Sara commented, "he probably doesn't want to leave his bed."

Exactly. Afterall, this happened in the bathroom, all of 10 feet away from his bed and with the oxygen on him.

"I guess it's not good that it happened, but there's a lesson there," Sara said. "The lesson is, he can't go home."

"Was May there when it happened?" Sara asked.

Yes. She whispered to me, "His oxygen level went down to 37%... I saw it."

"And that's not something you can inject into him?" Sara said. "You can't inject into him blood filled oxygen?"

Something like that wouldn't act fast enough to relieve his suffering; hence, it wasn't practical.

"Maybe he needs to be snowed?" Sara commented. "Is he on anti-anxiety medication?" Sara asked.

They were giving him antihistamines - The equivalent of Benadryl.

"Wait a minute," Sara said. "My grandmother was in her house, and they were giving her lorazepam - Ativan. And they won't give him benzos? I mean, it was explained to me that my grandmother was getting it for air hunger. Why aren't they giving that to Sam?"

I didn't know. It just seemed like more Ooga Booga (i.e., torture) to me.

I shook my head.

I'd never seen him lose control. He prided himself for always being "cool, calm and collected." Now, he was totally destabilized...

I shared with Sara that, before leaving, May had thoughtfully invited me to perform external Qi Gong on Sam. I wouldn't have suggested it, because, in that moment, it was my thought that what

Sam needed was well beyond anything that could be offered in Qi Gong.

Nevertheless, I did it; and when I did, there was feeling of activation of my crown chakra; instead, Qi flowed from Sam to my hand and then my solar plexus - The seat of emotions.

The night before, it felt like I was working to pull something out of his chest. The problem was, it induced coughing.

"So, now he's afraid," sara said. "He's petrified of coughing."

Yes. And for good reason.

It must have been some kind of strange bronchospasm that, intermixed with all that fibrosis in his lungs and chest cavity, combined to create the most horrible of human experiences.

"And you don't have any idea?" sara said. "It sounds like this is a very unusual situation, such that his lungs are not working like any other lungs you've probably ever looked at before. So, it might be hard for you to even imagine what's going on in there?"

"I mean, it's leather," she concluded. "It's like you were telling me before: It's basically one big scar - that's getting thicker and thicker."

Sara sighed.

"And that medicine attending was saying that in hospice they take away the oxygen," Sara said. "And he doesn't want the oxygen taken away. That's part of the suffering."

Sam's daughter Sandra called from Oakland. She wasn't aware of what happened at 5 PM, and I wasn't willing to tell her about it.

And neither did May. I think we both didn't want to share it. It was just too horrible to share with this young woman. A daughter.

"What does that feel like?" Sara asked.

The feeling of air hunger felt like the worst anxiety that you can imagine. Just remember what happened to me in the sweat lodge, when it turned me into a craze animal, scampering over people's arms and legs. Going out of my head. And I didn't even have a good reason for doing that. I just had the idea in my head that I was experiencing some air hunger. What Sam was going through was real - with an oxygen saturation of 37%!

"Is that what happened to all of those Jews who were in the gas chambers? For however many people - All going crazy in the end there?"

Yes.

"So, they basically tortured them," Sara commented. "Not just killed them, but tortured them."

Yes, it was more than whole-scale murder. It was whole-scale torture. The worst possible death imaginable.

On one occasion, I'd listened to a Nazi speak on the subject: He said that he and his comrades didn't care, because to them, Jews were just "vermin."

But their treatment towards the Jews was really so much worse than vermin. It was torture…

"If Sam was a dog," Sara commented, "you'd put the dog down."

She looked over at Cat Chow.

"If she gets like that... Well, it makes it easier to 'do the deed' with her…. Because what Sam's going through is torture."

Yes, two hours later and I was still shaking.

"I can't go through that again," I kept hearing in my head.

"And they didn't give him any Valium or anything?" She asked. "This person who just had this horrific near-death experience and they're not giving him anything but Benadryl? This is the time to give that to him. He's dying. It's like, 'What do you care if he gets addicted to it?'..."

I told sara about how it was that on my way home, I couldn't drive fast. I just couldn't get above 65 mph. Beyond that felt too jarring. I'm just so shaky and destabilized, just from listening to my friend's account of the experience.

Sara asked about May.

"Will she go home?" Sara asked.

I didn't think so. I think she was staying the night at the hospital.

"Is there a place for her to lie down?…"

There was a cot for her, but Sam's brother told me that she was mostly sleeping leaning over Sam's bedside…

When I considered how Sam had told me that the Palliative Care team was pressuring him to make a decision about leaving the hospital, I decided that from now on my attitude towards them was, "FU. Before you get Sam and his wife to make any decisions about discharge, you tell us exactly how you're going to keep them safe from an attack like this happening at home?" With an appropriate plan for him to be treated for those acute episodes. Because the need is going to arise.

I would tell them, "You have to convince us that you have an effective plan for this scenario. Because, to this point, you haven't

convinced me. The hospital hasn't even adequately responded to this kind of acute episode to this point. He is not stable for discharge."

How does this even happen? I thought. His wife witnessed Sam go to an oxygen saturation of 37%. She saw it.

And he's scared out of his mind, saying he can't experience that again. How will you prevent that from happening again?

And why was it OK for Sam to be admitted with no antibiotics and no respiratory treatments? How can he be admitted to the hospital that way and yet not be provided with the kinds of opioids and benzodiazepines to let him die in a more humane way?...

I confided to my friend, Reuben, about Sam's condition. That the continued process of fibrosis was probably cause his lungs to attach not just to his pleural cavity and chest wall, but also every other organ in his chest – So that the intense nausea he was experiencing with coughing was probably because his lungs were getting attached to his esophagus. Maybe the pain in his chest was in part because his lungs were getting attached to his pericardium and heart?

"I don't think we have any idea of the extent of the course of his disease," I said. "I don't think any of us could."

"Pain," Reuben responded. "And you feel like you have to cough all the time. And you can't get a good breath. And when you cough, your whole body explodes!"

Yeah, how did he know that? I thought.

"I had pneumonia," he said. "That's what it was like… You would get a coughing attack - Where you can't stop coughing?"

I described how his oxygen saturation went down to 37%.

"Right, because you can't breathe," he responded. "So, you're not getting oxygen in you. And anytime you try to take a deep breath, even a half breath, it makes you cough. Every time your lungs expand, it inflames it."

Reuben's description of it reminded me of Sam's description of nearly drowning in the ocean and being caught in the waves, and trying to surface to get a breath, but you can't because the next wave is crashing over you, and you're just taking that seawater into your throat, which is burning in your throat.

"Yep, that's exactly what it feels like," Reuben affirmed. "For two weeks I was bedridden with pneumonia. The year after we graduated. At the end of that summer, I got pneumonia, and I was in bed for two weeks.

"And I remember that. And it was a two-week fight to breathe. And anytime I coughed, I would cough up shit. And if I coughed too

much, my whole lungs would be inflamed and then I couldn't breathe. So, it was fighting against wanting to cough the whole time.

"And then if you go into the coughing spasms, it would take hours after that to calm your lungs down. To get any air in you."

That's the way Sam was after that attack. At 7 PM, he was still on that high flow oxygen.

"Was this his first attack? "Reuben asked.

No, but it did seem so much worse than any of the others.

"So, the other ones were warnings," Reuben responded. "This was the real thing."

"I don't know, Mike," Reuben concluded. "When I'm hurting or anything like that, I don't want anyone near me. I just want to go inward; I don't want to have to go outward. I mean, sometimes I think maybe Canada is right in allowing euthanasia - You give it to the choice of the patient. Maybe you should fly him to Canada?..."

CHAPTER THIRTY-ONE

Wednesday, August 13, 2025

Entering Sam's hospital room the following morning, May told me that (overnight) the covering doctors made plans for them to meet with the hospital hospice nurse.

"They came into the room and asked us if we wanted 'full comfort care'?" May said. "They kept saying, 'We could give you 'full comfort care. We could give you 'full comfort care.' We didn't know what that was, but it sounded good. We were just basically nodding our heads. I just figured he knew because he was the doctor..."

The hospice nurse was like an angel of mercy: When I said essentially that my friend wants to die as soon as possible so not to suffer anymore, she responded, 'Yes, that's exactly what your friend told us. You're all on the same page.'"

The hospital hospice nurse declared that she would do everything possible to see that adequate opioid medication was just a call to the nursing station away.

Furthermore, the hospice nurse indicated that she understood that this was not your typical hospice situation - That this was respiratory hospice, which required a heightened level of being able to act, so to be sure that the pain and suffering and anxiety was appropriately treated.

Everything she said was aligned with my heart.

I turned to Sam and asked Sam if he was OK with this? He said he was, and, with that, it was 'conversation closed': Hospital hospice was what we were going to do.

May signed some paperwork, and the nurse immediately initiation Sam was on a morphine drip at 5 mg per hour. So, whereas he was receiving perhaps 10 mg a day of morphine previously, now he was going to receive 120mg in a day…

"Did it seem to relieve him a little bit?" Sara asked.

Yes, it did.

Furthermore, the hospice nurse gave the family the permission to ask that morphine be administered to Sam if they felt he was suffering and needed more, as well as provided instructions for what to look for, suggesting signs of pain - such that if they felt that his wiggling his little toe was a sign that he was in pain, they could ask for more morphine.

"But does that mean that he's not conscious anymore?" Sara asked.

That was essentially what Sam wanted. He wanted to die. This will give him the means to do that comfortably.

"So, he's like my grandma was?" Sara asked. "Just out?"

That was my hope. He hadn't gone to that state when I left the room, but with 120 mg of morphine a day, for someone who was essentially opioid naïve, I hoped that's where he was going to be by the time I got back from Redding, where I was scheduled to give a talk as Northern California Pain Care Champion about opioid medications.

"So, now it's going to be how long his body can keep itself going with this kind of thing?" she asked. "Would this amount of morphine make it harder for him to breathe?"

Yes, it will lessen his respiratory drive.

"So, he'll probably slip away?"

Yes. Like he wanted to. Like he declared he needed to. They will let him die in peace.

"When is your best guess?" she asked.

I didn't know, I said. It was dependent the reserves of strength of Sam's body and how they responded to the medications. It was a complete wild card.

"Is he getting both benzodiazepines and morphine?" she asked.

Yes, no more Benadryl.

"I guess if you want the good stuff, you go with hospice," she responded. "When you're in hospice, all of this worry about addiction goes away…"

"I'm glad you were there to be there with him before he became snowed."

Yes, I would have stayed, but Sam asked that I do otherwise.

"I don't want to take you away from your work," he said. "Because you do important work..."

"And did his daughter come up?" Sara asked. "So, she got to say goodbye before he went slipping away?"

Yes, she was in the room when the hospice nurse talked with us.

"So, how are you feeling?"

I felt resolved. After seeing Sam after that attack yesterday and how terrified he looked, it was clear to me that the pain of living was worse than dying, and it was time.

"Like the way we felt when we let the process take place with Ini [our beloved dog]," Sara said. "Heartbroken, don't want it, but it's the only mercy..."

"Do May and Sandra understand?" she asked.

Yes, and among Sam's last words were his giving us permission to make mistakes.

"Because you're human," he said. "You're going to make mistakes..."

In any event, just like Ini, all of his systems were shutting down and going haywire. That's why nothing tasted good anymore. His time in this world for enjoying the fruits of the earth was over. They were turning off. The systems were going down. The body was saying that it was time to die. It's just what happens when it's your time. The system turns off and goes back to dust.

"Can I do anything for you?" Sara asked.

I didn't matter right now. It was just Sam who mattered - though I was aware that my circuits were getting crossed: I did make a mistake with a patient yesterday, but, fortunately, I was able to correct the mistake. Still, I was struggling; however, over the next two days, I was scheduled to give presentations in Redding and Sonora, which I can mostly do on cruise control. If I had patient responsibility, though, I would ask for leave…

"I'm wishing that I was more like you," Sara said, "and I had gone to Robert when he was there in the hospital. That will be a regret that I carry on with me for the rest of my life. And you won't have that regret when it comes to Sam. You'll know that he was important to you , and you were there for him."

Sara recalled how it was that during that time she was trying to get surgery for Cat Chow when it was found that she had that recurrence of cancer.

"Cat Chow needed me to help her, and I was doing that," she said. "So, I wasn't free to just get on a plane and go out to ROBERT. And his brother was telling me that ROBERT was comfortable, and I wanted to believe that. And my thoughts were on cat Chow. So, I prioritize cat chow over robert. Because cat chow was completely

dependent. She was my kid. She can't do it herself. And ROBERT was an adult. And he had his family members to help him. And I was still in shock from Ini being gone, and I didn't want cat chow to be gone. So, I made my decision.

"I believed that Robert was going to get home, and then I would come and visit him when he got home. I didn't think he wasn't ever going to get out of the hospital.

"And I do not believe that I'll make that decision again. Because then I was more trusting of hospitals. And now I've become very disillusioned about hospitals. Now I think, 'When someone I love goes to the hospital, I'm going to want to be there, so I can help with dealing with the hospital staff.'

"I don't have the clinical training that you do, so I won't be as knowledgeable as you are. Still, now I won't be, 'Oh, I'd rather see him at home, then be at the hospital.' From now on, I'll be in that hospital room, interacting with the doctors, and I'll actually be meeting somebody there in that room."

I thought about the regret I had regarding my mother and not staying with her after visiting her during that California society addiction medicine trip to San Diego.

"But your mom was not easy," sara asserted. "That's like an understatement. She was very difficult…"

Sara reminded me that, in Sam, I was losing not just a friend, but a brother, as defined in the Lakota culture.

"That's your brother," she said. "I mean, he's your brother!"

Yes, brother, teacher, father, guide, all rolled into one…

Wednesday night, after I got back from Redding and went to the hospital, there was no one with May.

May confided that she'd had disappointment, saying she left for an hour at about 1PM, and when she returned, Sam was no longer communicative, and she didn't think that that was going to happen.

"I just went home for an hour," she said. "I wasn't expecting that was going to be the last time I talked with Sam. I was expecting it to be that fast. I don't think he's ever going to wake up, and I would have liked to spend more time with him."

Whereas I was like, "I am OK with this. I don't want him to ever wake up. I don't want him to ever have to suffer again. I'm just fine with him passing. I'm just fine with that short conversation before I went away to Redding being our last…"

I told sara that talking with May reminded me of Sara's regrets about that last day in the park with Ini and how upset she was at herself for cutting that day short.

"That was the last day that Ini was happy," sara said. "She was so happy that you came to the park to join us. And then I left and came back and got everybody to come home."

"But maybe the fact that May was gone allowed Sam to let go," Sara added.

"But you don't think he's going to wake up again?" she asked. "If they stop the morphine, will he wake up?"

I don't think so. He might emit sounds here and there, but not wake up.

Indeed, when I returned from Redding, Sam was moaning, and his face looked tense, like he was having difficulty, his eyebrows furrowed; and even before I said anything, May was instructing the nurse to give Sam some IV Valium; and with that, his expression immediately relaxed…

Sara asked if Sam had any control on the morphine drip?

"Or is it just being automatically given to him?" she asked.

Not anymore, I said. With him in what amounted to a drug-induced coma that was essentially being left to us now.

And, yes, it was being automatically infused into him. When I left him, the morphine drip was set at 5 mg per hour; when I returned, it was 8mg per hour. At that rate and dose, it made for his being delivered 192 mg of morphine per day. Hence, for someone who was previously opiate naïve, I would say that would keep him quite snowed.

And I was happy that he was out, because I never wanted to see him the way he was yesterday again. I never wanted him to be terrified. I never wanted him to go through that kind of agony.

"So, now he's basically on a trip," Sara said. "He's tripping until he goes."

Yes. I just hope it's a happy trip. Because his body has been through enough. His "degrading", as he would say, has made it so he couldn't enjoy life. He couldn't enjoy the taste of any food that he used to like. It was all just "dust to dust." His was no longer a functioning machine. His time in this world is done. It's time to go to the next one and leave his dysfunctional mortal remains behind.

"Does May understand that?" Sara asked.

Yes. Indeed, when we talked this evening, she said as much.

"Sam was right," May had said. "He needed to be here where he could get immediate assistance for those attacks…"

"How long do you think he'll be coasting?" Sara asked.

I didn't know. I hadn't seen signs of Cheyne-Stokes (i.e., terminal) breathing.

Meanwhile, May had asked essentially the same exact question.

"Will I know if Sam passes if I go to sleep?" she'd asked.

I told her it was unlikely, being that he was no longer on any monitors.

"It could be that you'll wake up and he'll be gone," I'd said.

I indicated that I'd stay with her, but at about 11 PM, she indicated she was alright on her own, saying, "OK, I want to turn in. I'm pretty tired. I want to get some rest. I didn't get much rest last night…"

"What are you feeling?" Sara asked. "Can you reschedule your talk in Sonora… How would you feel if you weren't there when Sam passes away?"

I said that I would feel fine.

"It's over," I declared. "This taught me that our bodies are not meant to live forever. When it's time for you to die, they get messed up, and they could be a source of hell. And when it's a source of hell, it's time to move on."

"That was Ini," sara asserted. "She was in so much hell."

I asked why she felt that way.

"You didn't see the heart in her face," Sara responded. "Me and Ini shared this horrified look - when she couldn't breathe."

Yes, Sam's difficulty breathing was when I realized that I had to let him go. So, I was happy with the current situation. It has succeeded in keeping Sam from suffering like he did yesterday.

It was hard, though: For Sam, I think I feel pure love. And I think he felt that way about me, too. Yes, our relationship was a lot about fun - Skating, skiing, OneWheeling, sharing, thoughts, writing. But, at its core, was love.

"I think the Lakota call that 'cola'," Sara said. "You're a chosen brother – especially intellectually."

I didn't know that anybody was at Sam's intellectual level. "The wise man of metaphors", as I referred to him. He was in a class by himself.

"Yeah, but it was a brain that you could sound things off of."

Yes, I totally appreciated his brain. I will miss him, but not enough to want him around. Not after what he experienced yesterday…

"What's death like from pneumonia?" Sara asked.

It's described as the "old man's friend."

"Yeah, that's what people told us when my grandma B died," Sara said.

Still, where they weren't originally going to treat Sam with antibiotics, it does raise concerns about it contributing to an unpleasant delirium.

"So, you think this way is more merciful?" Sara asked. "Do you think he's on a trip and he's tripping."

I hope so. I hope that he was on a pleasant trip on morphine and benzodiazepines. Yeah, I wanted to think that he was on a pleasant trip - Without suffering.

"Did he seem calm?" She asked.

Yes, after they gave him the IV push of Valium; then he was calm, because an ease took hold of him; and I knew that he was no longer suffering. Not in any way.

"Did May also notice it?" Sara asked.

Yes, she and the nurse noted it.

"He needed the cocktail," Sara asserted.

Yes, the combination of opioid and benzodiazepine made the difference. It gave him that ease. And now it was, as sara had sang to her grandmother on her last night, time to "Row Row Row your boat gently down the stream…"

CHAPTER THIRTY-TWO

Thursday, August 14, 2025

I saw Sam on his OneWheel entering Jasmine's salon. I followed him inside, but then turned and walked out, feeling like I needed to give the two of them their time together.

But I changed my mind, because I wanted to hear what they said to each other, and turned to go back.

Then, I realized I was dreaming and pulled myself out of the dream...

Sitting up in bed, I considered the dream's meaning, especially with respect to a conversation with Sam some ten years ago:

After skating with my friend, Sam, we walked to the nearby Vietnamese restaurant for some refreshment. Seated at a booth we continued a philosophical discussion we'd been carrying on along the way. Then, Sam surprised me by asking how I envision heaven?

I demurred.

"Haven't given it much thought," I responded.

Indeed, I didn't think I'd given the subject any thought.

"Com'on," he said, prodding and laughing in his usual good-natured way. "You must have some concept of what it would be like."

Turning my head to the darkness outside the window, I opened my mind to the thought. And instead of white palace perched atop wafty clouds with a pearly gate in front, what registered was a vision of an angel that looked just like Jasmine!

I'd been fretting about the fact that Sam didn't seem to have a feeling or belief in the enduring nature of the soul and spirit, and just the other week, I confided that to Jasmine during my appointment with her…

I got up and drove to the hospital; however, as I was getting near, the oil light came on in my car. I knew that was bad, but I wanted to get to Sam.

I parked and went to Sam's room. Observing his breathing, I thought he would probably be around in the evening, and I could go to Sonora and deliver my in-service presentation and get back in time to have more time with Sam.

But how was I going to get to Sonora with the car in likely need of repairs?

Going back to the car, I checked the oil and found it was empty. Calling the mechanics at H&R Auto (whose services Sam had originally recommended to me), and spoke with Ray, who expressed concerns and strongly recommended against my driving to Sonora.

Ray told me to take the car into the shop but said they wouldn't be able to look at the car for a few hours because there were several cars ahead of me.

Calling Sara, she suggested that I get a government vehicle from work to use for the trip, and recalling that among Sam's final words was his saying my work was important, I put a quart of oil into the car (Having that quart of oil there was also at Sam's suggestion), and before leaving, went back to Sam and his family and let them know that I had to hurry off to the Transportation Office, but I'd be back after my talk.

May indicated that was all right and wished me good luck.

Before leaving, I humorously whispered the contents of the dream with Jasmine into Sam's ear…

Given the car trouble and last-minute government vehicle loaner, it looked like I was going to arrive late at Sonora. So, I called ahead to the clinic. Talking with the VA operator, she wrongly transferred me to a different call center than the Sonora VA. commented that she recognized my name and shared how it was that many patients would call her and ask for me and tell her what a great doctor I was.

When I called again, I got the same VA operator. A previous iteration of myself (The one that was possessed by cruel uncle) would have given this woman a hard time; but this one was guided by Sam, and I decided to give her a break, and be "cool, calm and collected" the way he lived. And the results were excellent: This lovely person apologized for her mistake, got me to the Clinical Director at Sonora, and even paid me a compliment to you, relaying that many of the

Veterans who she's interacted with, speak highly of me.

"Cool, calm and collected" is mostly the best way to be with people, I decided. It's what I kept telling myself when I was in this bind between the car and being late and getting to Sonora.

Be like Sam, I thought. Cool, calm and collected…

At the Sonora VA Clinic, I delivered the presentation; however, even though the subject matter was like second nature to me, it just felt like my delivery was off.

"I'm sorry if I'm a little preoccupied," I confided to those in attendance. "My best friend has been in the hospital…"

After the talk, I spoke with those in attendance, and they thanked me for coming out from Sacramento.

Then, just as I was making my way into Calaveras, I got the text from May, saying Sam had passed at 2:24 PM.

"It was faster than I thought" was my first reflection. I thought watching him breathing that morning, there wasn't Cheyne-Stokes yet, so I had enough time to deliver the presentation at Sonora and get back to Sam while he was still living.

I was wrong…

Stanley called me shortly after May texted about Sam's passing.

"I wanted to thank you for all you've done for me and May and Sandra and my whole family," he said. "Really appreciate it."

I asked if Sam passed peacefully?

"Yes, yes, he did," he responded.

I asked if the family was getting together?

"Not right now," he replied. "I think May needs some rest.… Sandra's gonna be with her, so I think she's going to process everything. It probably hasn't all hit her yet. but I will keep you informed about anything that happens with the family."

"Thank you for everything," he concluded. "Sam loved you. Really, he always talked about how he valued your friendship and your expertise, so thank you for everything."

I said I loved Sam, too…

Calling Sara about Sam's passing, she shared how it was that earlier in the morning when I told her that the oil light came on in the car and I was trying to figure out what to do about it, her first thought was, "Call Sam."

"Now, we're the elders," she declared...

I confided that I didn't think Sam's passing would be this quick – I thought I had time to present in Sonora and then get back in time to be with him before he passed.

"Are you sad you went?" Sara asked.

Yes and no. It's what Sam would have wanted, saying I did "important work"; however, I would have liked to be there.

"Were there other people there?" Sara asked.

Yes, May, Sandra, Stanley.

"Well, they had each other," she replied. "And Sam was already not conscious. And they were being supported by the medical staff in the hospital, so I think it was OK for it to be a family thing."

Yes, that was better.

"But you thought you'd be able to visit him?"

Yes, I thought that he was going to be alive into the evening. And now I was experiencing this emptiness in my heart, and I felt in need for some closure and just talking about Sam.

"When a light like this leaves this world," I said. "Well, I was filled with questions. Like how could for someone like Sam, they're not the throngs of friends and followers outside his hospital room door, waiting in a dirge and keeping up with the events surrounding his passing? Where were they?"

"Maybe they were like me, giving the people who were closer to him space to be with him," she said. "Because if I would have shown up, then it would've been a drag, and they would've felt like they had to be polite. Like it would've taken more than it gave, I think."

True. Nevertheless, it is my hope that when I die, there will be friends and followers outside my hospital room, waiting in a dirge. I wanted to leave behind students and disciples of energy medicine. That's what I want to be celebrated for when I leave this earth.

Sara sighed

"Your life…"

She broke off.

"I hear you, and I know this is something that's there's a need for you," she continued. "But it hurts me… I mean, it really… I don't know the word for it? It really makes me sad that you don't see that you're already making a difference in people's lives.

"I mean, you're already healing people. Like even with your conventional medicine. And what do I mean 'even'? With your life and what you do, every day you make a difference in somebody's life."

But there was a way that I wanted to make a difference. I wanted to advance the frontiers of energy medicine.

"Yes, but what I'm trying to say is that I hear that, but don't belittle what you've already contributed - What you already do. People already know that you helped them. You're already doing that.

"And I know there's a different modality that has helped you a lot and that you want to pursue. And that's admirable. And you're working on that. But regardless of where that path takes you, you're already helping people. You're already making a difference in people's lives.

"I mean, you've been doing it for 40 years! And when they create a vaccine for cancer, which looks like they're really working on and getting somewhere with… Well, even if you're not officially recognized, you're at the root of it.

"So, you've already made a contribution. And I know you want to make more contributions, and you're working on them, and you will make more contributions. And you've already done it.

"And I'm sorry you missed this time to see Sam pass away, and you feel like you don't have closure because you weren't there when he passed. It sounds a little bit like what May was going through yesterday when she said that she missed the moment that he drifted out of consciousness."

Yes, I would have liked to scan him energetically.

"Is that something that May would have been comfortable with?" she asked.

Perhaps, but, in truth, I had been refraining from doing that with Sam since he drifted out of consciousness, because there were always members of his family in the room, and I didn't want this to be about me - I wanted this to be about him and them.

"Yeah," she affirmed…

I told Sara I was perplexed about Sam passing without the lines of people waiting outside his door, doing a dirge because this wonderful extraordinary human being was leaving this world. I saw it before with that medical school professor, Dr. Harvey, who I even didn't like, yet there were all those medical students outside his door, and I didn't think he nearly deserved that as much as Sam. Dr. Harvey wasn't anything near the professor that Sam was.

"I don't think it was important to Sam," she said. "He was a private person. He had his ski students. Otherwise, he was a private person."

Still, it all left me wanting to cry out, "Where are the lines? Where is the love? Where is the appreciation?"

"You are the line!" Sara declared. "You are the line! You are the love! You are the appreciation!"

But it's crazy that I'm all there is, I responded.

"It's OK!" she asserted. "It's OK. Everybody is fine. It's OK. You are the line. You carry that torch…"

EPILOGUE

[Matisse] challenges the conventional understanding of any artist's "late" years as an inevitable tapering off. Here, we see a blossoming, a relentless drive to experiment in new mediums and a radical simplicity that only a lifetime of making could achieve."
~ Emily LaBarge, New York Times

Saturday, August 16, 2025

I woke up to a vision of Jasmine walking hand-in-hand into the "great beyond" with a shadowy silhouette possessing Sam's general build and physique. It looked like the figure from Henri Matisse's Icarus…

"The dreams are showing you that there's something there," a friend (Jajuan) asserted. "'Don't worry. I'm in good hands. I'm in heaven. Don't worry because I'm in heaven or the afterlife or whatever we should call it.'

"Because everyone has, even if they don't believe in the hereafter within them, they do have an idea of light and energy, and they will naturally be drawn to that when their soul is leaving their body. They will just naturally go there. And they'll be support for them there to guide them. For those who do not have what they expect and want, they do have helpers.

"I've had a recurring vision since I was a little kid. To me that is a form of transition, and it's definitely nature related, it's like a meadow with a white deer, and I've had that dream forever. And I feel like that's a little part of my soul in a beautiful valley, with incredible nature and wildflowers and deer and the smells are all there. And by the time that I'm ready to leave my body, I might have

a different feel for what it might be like, but I have a lot of confidence and peace about it. I'm not worried about it at all, because I believe in our ancestors, and I know that it's energy. It's light and energy and peace and joy to the ecstasy of light and joy.

"And I know they'll be guides that will be helping. And I believe, depending on the mental state of those who are passing, there is always going to be a middle area of comfort to them and self-awareness for their souls.

"So, they'll be guides for them. I think we all have guides. And whether it's Christianity or Buddhism, I think it's all fabulous; I believe there's just people to guide us in this life. There's some of the teachings."

"And I just think we're all connected in the same soul," she concluded, "and that we all connect into one. We are spirits having a human experience, so that we can be even further in light..."

Sam's disease brought me to my knees: When it was time for him to pass, the only thing that mattered to me was getting the opioids and benzodiazepines into his system to give him relief; and I had essentially no interest in performing BioEnerQi with him.

About a month after his passing (on Saturday, September 20, 2025 at Sam's Celebration of Life ceremony), Sam's humor was in full display.

"Sam was joyful and funny, and so appreciative of the blessings of life," the pastor began. "When I went to Sam and asked him how he would like to how have his memorial service observed, he said, 'Well, I think it would be really neat if you put my ashes in a piñata and gave everybody a turn to take a whack at it."

In response, I couldn't stop laughing.

That was quintessential Sam, I thought.

"As well as cry over Sam no longer being here, you also have permission to laugh, for there is so much about Sam that was joyful and funny and so appreciative of the blessings of life," the pastor continued. "I think Sam understood that even the most difficult challenges in life offered opportunities to grow. As a pasture, I think it's important to set our remembrance of Sam in God's will for eternal hope. And I really mean that in a universal way. As an affirmation for the many religious traditions that speak to truth. Because I know to all of those who knew Sam, there was much about him that we would say, indeed, that reflected God's spirit of concern and love and generosity. In that regard, I think that Sam was very much connected

to the heart of God in so many ways. Because he lived his life and held his relationships with remarkable heart and spirit and love.

"So, today we share our sorrow, and we hope that it is made lighter, knowing that we are gathered together in community. Our presence to one another, indeed brings comfort. That the word spoken by many of us today will reflect the feelings of us all. And that somehow we feel the presence of God in this place that finds us together in love.

"And I hope that through it all, Sam truly knows how much he was loved and continues to be so. Sam was blessed with so much life by his family and his many friends. We thank you for the love through which Sam was nurtured and sustained through family and friends. We thank you for the way that Sam was supportive in life and provided kindness and caring towards others. Oh God, behind us together in our love for Sam. Bring comfort to our souls and remind us that as much as we wish Sam was still here with us, Sam was released from his weakening physical condition and immersed in your eternal peace.

"As well as cry over Sam no longer being here, you also have permission to laugh, for there is so much about Sam that was joyful and funny and so appreciative of the blessings of life. I think Sam understood that even the most difficult challenges in life offered opportunities to grow…"

Photos of Sam taken throughout his life were shared, and I was surprised that I didn't find him as handsome when he was young as I did later in life, and it seemed he was just one of those individuals who grew more handsome with age. Indeed, in the photos taken when he was younger, he looked more like he a mild-mannered, committed scientist, with a good sense of humor, just like he'd described himself, and a typical, friendly, nonthreatening "model minority" Asian. And not that Sam was threatening to anyone (He was the last person in the world like that!) but he did have strong views and opinions: He cared about people and the state of the world to his bones! When I shared his humanitarian side in my eulogy, my voice roared his thoughts against persecution, just as his words on the subject still roared head in my head.

Still, when it comes to my enduring image of Sam, it's the joy-filled ski sensei, effortlessly flying down a mountain slope, with snow like angel dust, magically kicked up and trailing behind him...

Now, I'm going to come clean and tell you that the image of my friend (as a dark silhouette in that second vision with Jasmine) shook me and wasn't at all what I imagined as "heaven" or the hereafter or the "great beyond."

So, on Yom Kippur, Thursday, October 2, 2025, when our temple rabbi invited members of the congregation who were grieving to stand before the Torah scroll (the holiest object of the Jewish religion), I thought about Sam and his appreciation for members of the Jewish community and Jewish traditions and decided to take engage the opportunity. And standing there, what I saw on my mind's eye was an exquisitely beautiful crystalline blue-black lattice with light running all through and around it, not unlike what I'd seen in that image of Sam moving away with Jasmine.

Then, I thought, "Sam, can you give me a sign?" and, in turn, I felt energy all over and especially inside of me, which I'd only experienced the once when Sam commented about his experiencing that way.

And backing away from the Torah, I was left thinking that being a spirit was great, but I could imagine that at a certain point you get tired of just existing in all that exquisite darkness, and in spite of all the suffering and struggles and pain that you knew in your previous iteration living in the physical plane before you went back to the spirit world, you think to yourself, "Well, I think I can handle it", and do it again after all, maybe even sooner than I would have thought. Indeed, I'm reminded of something Sam told me about love and taking chances in life:

"Love at first site is about what attracts us," he said. "That's what makes people take on these really incredible endurance tests. That's what makes them conquer Antarctica. If a person really did study it too much, they probably wouldn't do it, because they'd say, 'I could get frostbite. I can lose my toes. I could lose my nose. My ears.' All of a sudden, you go, 'You know what, I'm not gonna do it.'

"But people don't think that. They just think of all the wonderful things, and the adrenaline they have, and 'It's can be so cool', and 'I'll really see how strong I really am', and say, 'Okay, I'm going to go for it. And no one's gonna stop me.'

"So, we've got all these flaws, or else we'd do everything perfect! But then we wouldn't learn anything. So, imperfection makes us perfect, so to speak..."

Finally, when I look back and consider my efforts to help Sam with Qi Gong, I wonder that I wasn't too strong in my belief that it could help him? In my defense, my experience with Sam had been marked by pushing me to the limits of my ability with external Qi Gong and then rising to them, and I was hoping that that pattern would happen here; I was endeavoring to use Qi Gong to help Sam when there were not other options available to him for his interstitial lung disease; and I'd just come off if significant success treating patients with problems of long COVID, which has been seen as, in part, an autoimmune process. However, in retrospect, in many ways helping Sam was not unlike the efforts I described thirty years ago to help Ethel with her cancer. Back then, based on my years of cancer research, I mainly saw the development of cancer as a manifestation of a breakdown in communication between single cells and the body as a whole. This is based on the following: Each cell of the body is there to promote the general welfare of the person; each has self-suicide pathways (called apoptosis) to activate when things go wrong, so that in response to being exposed to carcinogenic toxins and mutation-causing free radicals, the cell turns on the self-suicide programs, so to self-destruct and thereby protect the organism as a whole. The gene most responsible for activating this self-destruct process is called 'p53.' It's only when genes like p53 are mutated that these cells undergo malignant and become cancerous. Indeed, p53 is mutated in a majority of human malignancies.

However, even when mutated, I know from firsthand experience that p53 mutations still possess some residual apoptotic function that can be triggered and to facilitate cellular self-destruction; and I believe Qi Gong can trigger this reaction in cancer cells.

"You're not incorrect," a Qi Gong master responded. "Mostly, my instructors in Beijing talked about how they had to get the immortal aspect to go dormant, so that the cancer can turn back into a regular cell, so it can slough off, and the mass shrink and go from solid to liquid and disperse."

"So, you're correct," he concluded. "It's just that when you're talking about cancer and telling cancer cells to lay down their lives for the general good, it's like asking a contentious five-year old to give up his favorite toy because that's the better thing to do – And that doesn't always go well."

And it didn't "go well" for Ethel with her cancer; and then, it didn't "go well" for Sam with his Interstitial Lung Disease.

In spite of this, I don't intend to quit, and in the future, in the spirit of my beloved friend, I plan to press forward and perform the scientific investigations to define the therapeutic limits of external Qi Gong, including in the treatment of cancer and autoimmune diseases, just as Sam advised me.

"Look, the implications of all these things you're doing are just incredible," he told me. "But you have to be realistic and practical, otherwise you're not going to progress..."

Still, the passing of my friend is a hard pill to swallow, "so to speak", as he would say. I tried as hard as I could to help him, until I had to let go.

And it pains me now to think that my efforts might have been misguided, and he was right all the time, and mostly went along with my efforts because it was a way that he could continue to help and guide me, even as he was facing the most difficult days of his life…

Talking with an insightful nurse, she referred to Sam as "patient zero", who I could compare everyone else, in the way of what worked and what didn't work - What conditions would benefit from Qi Gong, and what needed conventional medicine.

Losing Sam has left me more serious, solemn, pragmatic. It certainly feels like I'm not looking at things with the same rose-colored glasses that I used to. Indeed, when it comes to the kind of love that Sam talked about that made people conquer the unknown, it doesn't feel like I have as much of that anymore.

So, there it is: In the end, you have here what Sam regarded as the promise and limits of this approach, though I'm sure he'd tell you to consider them "with a grain of salt"...

A year after Sam's passing, I was invited to present my Qi Gong research at the 2026 Science of Tai Chi & Qigong conference at Harvard University Medical School. There, Dr. Wayne Jonas (former Director of the Office of Alternative Medicine at the National Institutes of Health from 1995 to 1999) talked about Salutogenesis, which is the movement towards restoring health after illness.

And listening, I felt Salutogenesis was exactly what BioEnerQi had done for the participants of the Long Covid-Qi Gong study, because long COVID essentially amounted to a person having gone through an acute illness (COVID) and afterwards being "stuck", so that their symptoms of illness were not resolving, and it took BioEnerQi to initiate the process of moving towards health.

However, in Sam's case, the disease wasn't done with him the way it was for those long COVID folks. Yes, long COVID is felt to have an element of autoimmunity, but I don't think it's active and aggressive the way that it was with Sam's condition. In the case of those long COVID folks, the pathogenesis process had essentially sputtered out and now the system just needed to be rebooted in order to move in the direction towards health. Hence, their systems were ready for salutogenesis. In Sam's case, however, the pathogenesis process was still charging full-steam ahead! Hence, what Sam needed was something entirely different than the long COVID folks: He needed a therapeutic intervention that would activate the apoptotic mechanisms of those autoimmune cells, as well as set in motion fibrolytic pathways to reverse all that scarring throughout his lungs and other parts of his system, and that didn't happen!

Like I said, I haven't given up on the possibility that BioEnerQi is capable of this; but, certainly, to date, I haven't been able to break that code.

"To me, BioEnerQi is like giving a patient oxygen," participant from the Long COVID-Qi Gong study, Ruth, declared. "To give them more of what their body needs, so that their body can do what it needs to do if it's going to heal. And sometimes it needs more time."

Yes, and time ran out…

Questions do remain within the Post-Study Qi Gong group as to Sam's "belief" in the process.

"I wonder how much of an impact that any form of healing has if we don't have a belief in the healing?" Rosa commented. "I think Sam reached a point where we weren't sure whether or not he was believing that he was healing with Qi Gong?

"And at the beginning [of the Long COVID-Qi Gong study], I didn't know, either. But when I realized I was healing, I believed in the healing. So, I healed.

"I could have just as easily said, 'No, this is not helping me', and then, I think it wouldn't have helped.

"I just believe that we control part of that – part of the healing process – and getting the cells to manifest getting better."

"If an organ gets too diseased and is already dying," Ruth added, wisely, "I don't know how possible it is to heal it. We're really not in control…"

Talking with my cousin, Jerry (who is also active in Biofield Therapy) about my efforts to help Sam, then losing him and regretting that I'd been unrealistically hopeful, Jerry offered words of sympathy and advice.

"I don't think it hurts to try," he began, "but it's just hard to learn to not be attached to the results - Just to know that you can only do what you do, and you kind of 'Give it up to God' and see what happens."

In retrospect, I was obviously coming off of the success of the Long COVID-Qi Gong study; and, as stated, long COVID is thought to have a significant autoimmune component, so I was hopeful that this success would carry over to Sam: That I would connect energetically with Sam, and effect a communication with his

autoimmune cells; and help them recognize they were harming Sam; and what they needed to do was self-destruct, as well as his body activating mechanisms tap into the body's ability to reverse all of this fibrosis.

And his disease didn't respond like that at all. And hence, Sam was likely right all along to be pragmatic.

"What part bothers you?" my cousin asked. "Do you feel like you over-promised and under-delivered?"

Yes, that's it: Despite all this being based on theory (and there being no reason to anticipate a successful outcome), I was so hoping it would help that I became too invested in it.

"Well, that is really hard - because it is your best friend!" my cousin correctly asserted. "I mean, of course you want to help him. And also, it's really normal to want to give somebody hope. And I think it's pretty cool on his part that he's like, 'Hey, sure, we can do this, but I'm not going to put too much stock in it.' I mean, his intuition kind of knew that it wasn't going to help, but I'm sure that you gave him comfort, and he appreciated it as part of your friendship - That you were trying to give what you could to him."

"And he probably recognized your disappointment, too," he acknowledged, "but it's just a normal human thing."

"I mean, I tell you," he continued, "in my prayer ceremonies, I've had a number of people come to me in wheelchairs. And I'll never forget this one kid who was wheeled in on this portable hospital bed. And I just wanted to help so bad. I mean, I've never had anybody in my services get up out of a wheelchair and be like, 'Hallelujah, I'm healed.' I've seen miracles happen, but not that. And this kid… Well, I knew his parents had done everything they could with this kid as far as conventional, holistic, and everything; and I was just another step on the path; and I just so wanted that kid to get up off of that portable hospital bed that they wheeled him in on. But he didn't. And nobody that has ever come to me in a wheelchair has ever gotten out of it.

"In fact, there's a number of people that I know of, including a very close friend of mine, who came to my ceremonies hoping for healing and actually ended up dying - like a few days later. But dying really peacefully, like able to finally just let go. And their death, as it was reported to me by their friends and loved ones, was easy, peaceful, not painful. So really, I took that on as a healer, as well, even though I wanted them to have a miracle recovery.

"So, it's a hard line not to trip over when you have to try and remain neutral; but yet you want something for somebody else, and

you want it also for your own ego to say, 'Hey, what I'm doing really works'."

"It's just mysterious," he concluded. "It's really tough."

Yes, Sam had always led me to elevate my practice. Before Sam, I was still doing the Bioenergy that Dr. Rind taught me; even though Master Chou had taught me external Qigong, I wasn't there. Then, that one day that I was working with Sam on a problem of headache changed everything: I knew I was capable of more, and after a long convoluted internal Qi Gong self-practice, it happened, and I undeniably performed external Qi Gong for the first time.

It took that desire to help Sam to elevate my practice. And I was hoping that that same desire might elevate my practice of external Qi Gong again and make it possible for me to help Sam overcome his terminal illness and get those autoimmune cells to activate their apoptotic mechanisms and self-destruct, instead of taking Sam's life. And, lo and behold, that didn't happen, and now I was without my friend.

"Well, you know what?" my cousin responded. "That practice, that whole thing might actually have elevated your practice, even though it didn't succeed with Sam. It's possible that your effectiveness and your abilities went up a notch, even though, sadly, it didn't help your great friend."

"In any event, I hope the lesson was to go into this without ego," he concluded.

Yes, as he said, from a "neutral state."

"It's not easy," he declared. "But, yes, that is the goal. But we're all human…"

Some twenty-five years earlier, on the night after my cherished friend, Ethel, died of cancer, my then guide, Elizabeth, reached out to me.

"I just had the feeling like I should call," she'd said. "How is Ethel?"

After listening to me recount the previous night's events, she responded, "Mike, the intricacies and interweavings of the fabric of the Universe never cease to amaze me... Here's Ethel - In her last moments in this world - Giving you a piece of her heart - To help mend your heart..."

"Mike, it was never about Ethel," she concluded. "It was about you! Ethel's life was over - She was going to die - It's you who gets to go on living..."

All these thoughts also apply to Sam: Sam knew he was going to die, and with what strength and intellect he had left, he was going to

experientially guide me to realistically take the study of BioEnerQi into the future.

About a year after Sam's passing, I had the opportunity to go whale watching in Monterrey Bay. I knew I had problems of seasickness; but whereas the worst part of Sam's suffering had been the gnawing feeling of nauseousness in his stomach, I felt even more motivated to have that experience: So to be closer to my friend, and suffer what he'd suffered.

Casting off for a four-hour trip, the seasickness came on relatively quickly; and, unlike Sam, after I'd thoroughly ejected the contents of my stomach, the nausea mostly released me; as though it gave me mercy, and let up, so to allow me to engage in the experience; and in the end, it felt like I'd conquered something and, as usual, had Sam to be grateful for it: Because the fact that he'd gone through that difficulty and done it with a smile and grace, he'd provided me an example to emulate.

"And did you feel you had that grace?" Steve asked when I shared the story.

Yeah, I replied. Yeah, when people on the boat would come and ask how I was doing, I'd just smile back at them and say, "I'm doing great. I really appreciate being out here and seeing the whales."

And it was great. The day was beautiful, and I saw amazing things that I could have never imagined: Seals keeping up with dolphins and swimming with them, side-by-side; humpback whale calves repeatedly "breaching" (jumping out of the water) at the urgings of their mothers; and the largest creatures on earth (blue whales and fin whales) looking magnificent, as they swam in proximity with one another.

And I'd done it all from the very bow of the ship, because I'd been told that was the best place for viewing the whales, in what I imagined would be a once in a lifetime experience that I would have never engaged in had I let my previous experiences with seasickness guide me.

And it made me happy – because I'd done something hard, faced down something I was afraid of, and came out better because of it.

And I'd accomplished it in a way that showed I'd learned from my friend; and rather than fall back on learned behavior from my upbringing, I'd been "cool, calm and collected" (as Sam would say of himself), treating the experience with a sense of humor and a smile.

"It's always good to 'purge' yourself of life's stresses and 'dive' into nature," Sam's cousin, John, texted when I shared the adventure.

I recalled my Qi Gong instructor, Paul Mok, who told me about how it was that when he was initiated into Qi Gong, he just kept vomiting and vomiting, and explaining it as 'purging' himself of a lot of turbid Qi that had been trapped in his system. I felt it was the same for me in my whale adventure, and now I was ready to embrace more adventures.

"It must have been a 'whale' of a time," John wrote, concluding his text. "Sorry for the puns – It's a Sam thing."

That it is, I agreed...

In a final vision, Sam came to me in a dream to teach me how to play an ancient Asian wooden musical instrument. With its hourglass-shape and many grooves, the instrument looked not unlike a Janggu. To play it, Sam patiently instructed me to use a delicate wooden stick (like a *bachi)* and tap between the grooves, starting at the top and sequentially moving downward. I tried, but my technique was too mechanical. So, Sam took the stick and demonstrated: It was tap, tap, double tap, tap, tap, and his flowing technique produced a vibration that not only sent the instrument pleasantly humming, but the vibration extended to the stick, as well.

Then, with a flick of the wrist, Sam effortlessly sent the stick spinning and vibrating off into the universe forever…

ABOUT THE AUTHOR

Michael Yanuck MD PhD is a physician-scientist whose groundbreaking research at the National Institutes of Health was the basis for an FDA-approved vaccine for cancer. Following a traumatic leg injury, he trained in Bioenergy and Qi Gong, introduced Energy Medicine techniques at the National Center for Complementary and Integrative Health, and worked with Chi Gong Masters who were part of the President's Executive Committee on Alternative Medicine. For his work with Veterans in the VA Innovation Accelerator-Qi Gong project, he received the 2023 Science of Tai Chi & Qigong Award from Harvard University and co-led the University of California-Davis Long COVID-Qi Gong project, providing hope to those with long COVID.

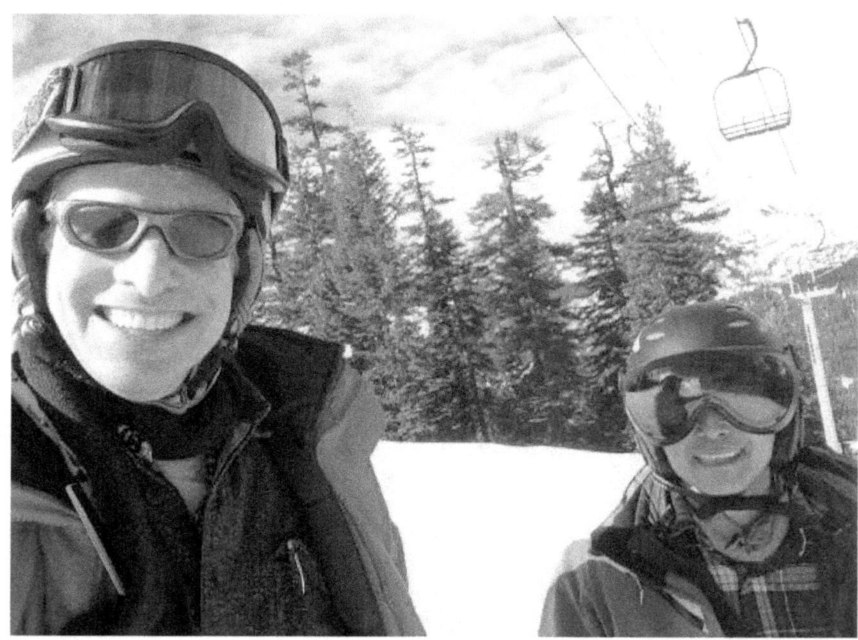

www.ingramcontent.com/pod-product-compliance
Lightning Source LLC
LaVergne TN
LVHW020046110826
845155LV00029B/643

* 9 7 8 1 9 4 6 6 0 0 4 8 6 *